T0202118

Published and forthcoming Oxford Handbooks

Oxford Handbook for the Foundation Programme 4e
Oxford Handbook of Acute Medicine 3e
Oxford Handbook of Anaesthesia 4e
Oxford Handbook of Applied Dental Sciences
Oxford Handbook of Cardiology 2e
Oxford Handbook of Clinical and Healthcare Research
Oxford Handbook of Clinical and Laboratory Investigation 3e
Oxford Handbook of Clinical Dentistry 6e
Oxford Handbook of Clinical Diagnosis 3e
Oxford Handbook of Clinical Examination and Practical Skills 2e
Oxford Handbook of Clinical Haematology 4e
Oxford Handbook of Clinical Immunology and Allergy 3e
Oxford Handbook of Clinical Medicine—Mini Edition 9e
Oxford Handbook of Clinical Medicine 10e
Oxford Handbook of Clinical Pathology
Oxford Handbook of Clinical Pharmacy 3e
Oxford Handbook of Clinical Rehabilitation 2e
Oxford Handbook of Clinical Specialties 10e
Oxford Handbook of Clinical Surgery 4e
Oxford Handbook of Complementary Medicine
Oxford Handbook of Critical Care 3e
Oxford Handbook of Dental Patient Care
Oxford Handbook of Dialysis 4e
Oxford Handbook of Emergency Medicine 4e
Oxford Handbook of Endocrinology and Diabetes 3e
Oxford Handbook of ENT and Head and Neck Surgery 2e
Oxford Handbook of Epidemiology for Clinicians
Oxford Handbook of Expedition and Wilderness Medicine 2e
Oxford Handbook of Forensic Medicine
Oxford Handbook of Gastroenterology & Hepatology 2e
Oxford Handbook of General Practice 4e

Oxford Handbook of Genetics
Oxford Handbook of Genitourinary Medicine, HIV, and Sexual Health 2e
Oxford Handbook of Geriatric Medicine 2e
Oxford Handbook of Infectious Diseases and Microbiology 2e
Oxford Handbook of Key Clinical Evidence 2e
Oxford Handbook of Medical Dermatology 2e
Oxford Handbook of Medical Imaging
Oxford Handbook of Medical Sciences 2e
Oxford Handbook of Medical Statistics
Oxford Handbook of Neonatology 2e
Oxford Handbook of Nephrology and Hypertension 2e
Oxford Handbook of Neurology 2e
Oxford Handbook of Nutrition and Dietetics 2e
Oxford Handbook of Obstetrics and Gynaecology 3e
Oxford Handbook of Occupational Health 2e
Oxford Handbook of Oncology 3e
Oxford Handbook of Operative Surgery 3e
Oxford Handbook of Ophthalmology 3e
Oxford Handbook of Oral and Maxillofacial Surgery
Oxford Handbook of Orthopaedics and Trauma
Oxford Handbook of Paediatrics 2e
Oxford Handbook of Pain Management
Oxford Handbook of Palliative Care 2e
Oxford Handbook of Practical Drug Therapy 2e
Oxford Handbook of Pre-Hospital Care
Oxford Handbook of Psychiatry 3e
Oxford Handbook of Public Health Practice 3e
Oxford Handbook of Reproductive Medicine & Family Planning 2e
Oxford Handbook of Respiratory Medicine 3e
Oxford Handbook of Rheumatology 3e
Oxford Handbook of Sport and Exercise Medicine 2e
Handbook of Surgical Consent
Oxford Handbook of Tropical Medicine 4e
Oxford Handbook of Urology 3e

OXFORD MEDICAL PUBLICATIONS

Oxford Handbook of Integrated Dental Biosciences

Oxford Handbook of
Integrated Dental Biosciences

Second Edition

Professor Hugh Devlin
Professor in Restorative Dentistry, University of
Manchester, UK

Dr Rebecca Craven
Senior Lecturer in Dental Health, University of
Manchester, UK

OXFORD
UNIVERSITY PRESS

OXFORD
UNIVERSITY PRESS

Great Clarendon Street, Oxford, OX2 6DP,
United Kingdom

Oxford University Press is a department of the University of Oxford.
It furthers the University's objective of excellence in research, scholarship,
and education by publishing worldwide. Oxford is a registered trade mark of
Oxford University Press in the UK and in certain other countries

© Oxford University Press 2018

The moral rights of the authors have been asserted

First Edition published in 2002

Published in the United States of America by Oxford University Press
198 Madison Avenue, New York, NY 10016, United States of America

British Library Cataloguing in Publication Data
Data available

Library of Congress Control Number: 2017955323

ISBN 978–0–19–875978–2

Printed and bound in Turkey by Promat

Foreword

Contemporary clinical teaching and learning in dentistry and other health professions now integrates the biosciences with clinical scenarios. This *Oxford Handbook of Applied Dental Sciences* is, however, the first that provides a format to support this style of learning.

Hugh Devlin and Rebecca Craven have a vast experience of teaching and learning in dentistry and have been at the forefront of advances in this integration. Understanding the relevance of the non-clinical science to the clinical practice that it underpins is now known to provide much more effective learning. This integration enables deep learning. It stimulates interest in the biosciences for the clinical learner and its application becomes more meaningful.

Hugh Devlin is a successful teaching and research enthusiast. He has taught undergraduates and postgraduates at the University of Manchester for over 35 years and his depth and breadth of experience could not be more appropriate for the development of this book. He is a respected clinical academic with over one hundred scientific publications many of which explore the link between basic dental science and their clinical application. Hugh received the IADR Distinguished Scientist Award (2011) for Research in Prosthodontics and Implants.

Rebecca Craven worked in general dental practice and community and hospital dentistry before spending over 25 years in successful university research and teaching. Rebecca, like Hugh, has vast experience in and a passion for teaching and learning and could not be better placed to produce this book. Her studying for the award of 'Fellowship in Dental Surgery' required returning to bioscience study after several years of clinical practice and this sparked a lifelong passion to integrate the two disciplines. Rebecca now leads postgraduate Masters programmes in both research and Dental Public Health, a discipline in which she is an NHS Consultant. She also leads the first year of the undergraduate dental programme. Integrating bioscience with clinical care and seeking to apply, appropriately, the best evidence, is at the heart of the University of Manchester Dentistry programmes and of this book.

This book is truly 'applied' and presents the bioscience as clinically relevant as possible, with a separate sections detailing the relevant clinical application and putting the science into context. This book therefore supports contemporary methods of teaching where students study a subject based on a clinical scenario. Hugh Devlin and Rebecca Craven have presented a 'systems' approach by describing how the different major organs work, what happens with disease, and how this affects the patient's dental treatment. Rather than discuss sections on pharmacology, histology, epidemiology, and public health, these subjects are woven throughout the text and referred to where their use is most relevant.

The first edition of this book was edited by the late Professor Crispian Scully and had separate sections on physiology, pathology, anatomy, and the rest. This second edition integrates the topics and focuses more closely on their clinical relevance so that readers will want to supplement their reading of this handbook from other texts, especially for detailed anatomy and cell biology. This book will be an invaluable resource for dental students and dentists studying for higher qualifications after graduation.

Paul Coulthard
BDS MFGDP(UK) MDS FDSRCS FDSRCS(OS) PhD
Dean of the School of Dentistry at the University of Manchester
and Professor of Oral and Maxillofacial Surgery

Preface

Our aim is to provide a pocket book of bioscience which is tailored to the needs of dental students. Our approach has been to provide knowledge that is relevant to clinical dental practice and is up-to-date. We want clinicians to reflect on the biological principles and mechanisms, which we hope will encourage deep learning. Science is essential to understand the signs and symptoms of any patient's disease and the clinician-scientist will be able to offer clear explanations when proposing treatment options to a patient.

Most undergraduate programmes now include some early introduction to dentistry alongside biosciences, but until now that change has not been reflected in textbooks. We aim is to bridge this gap and show directly the relevance of the biology to the clinician.

The previous handbook on this subject, the *Oxford Handbook of Applied Dental Sciences*, edited by the late Professor Crispian Scully, had separate sections on physiology, pathology, anatomy, and the rest. This new handbook seeks to integrate the topics and focus more closely on their clinical relevance so readers will want to supplement their reading of this handbook from other texts, especially for detailed anatomy and cell biology. The thirteen chapters lead the reader through the major body systems. In most cases, a one page opening is a succinct summary of a topic, enriched by diagrams and illustrations.

The authors have many decades of experience in clinical dentistry and learning and teaching where we have aspired to an integrated and evidence-based approach. The Oxford Handbook format is ideally suited to the dental undergraduate and has proved very popular and practical for students. It is also hoped that clinicians who are seeking to revise their understanding of biosciences or are preparing for higher clinical examinations may find this a useful starting point.

Hugh Devlin
Rebecca Craven
2017

Acknowledgements

The authors would like to acknowledge the help of Mr Daniel Wand at the University of Manchester who gave much assistance with many of the diagrams.

Contents

Symbols and abbreviations *xi*

1	Oral cavity and gut	1
2	Temporomandibular joint and surrounding musculature	39
3	Oral mucosa, saliva, and speech	65
4	Bone	85
5	Liver	111
6	Kidneys and chronic renal disease	133
7	Diabetes	149
8	The respiratory system	169
9	Heart and blood supply	187
10	Blood	207
11	Immune system	231
12	Central nervous system	257
13	Endocrine system	287

Index *305*

Symbols and abbreviations

&	and
=	equal to
×	multiply
α	alpha
β	beta
γ	gamma
κ	kappa
↑	increased
®	registered trademark
ACE	angiotensin converting enzyme
ACH	acetaldehyde
ACS	acute coronary syndrome
ACTH	adrenocorticotrophic hormone
APTT	activated partial thromboplastin time
ADCC	antibody dependent cellular cytotoxicity
ADJ	amelodentinal junction
ADP	adenosine diphosphate
ADS	anatomic dead space
AGE	advanced glycation end product
ALL	acute lymphoblastic leukaemia
ALP	alkaline phosphatase
ALT	alanine aminotransferase
AML	acute myeloid leukaemia
ACE	angiotensin converting enzyme
ANP	atrial natriuretic hormone
APC	antigen presenting cell
ARB	angiotensin receptor blockers
ASA	American Society of Anaesthesiologists
AST	aspartate aminotransferase
ATP	adenosine triphosphate
ATP	adenosine triphosphate
AV	atrioventricular
BMI	body mass index
BP	blood pressure
BSE	bovine spongiform encephalitis
CCK	cholecystokinin

CPG	central pattern generator
CHD	coronary heart disease
CIED	cardiovascular implantable electronic device
CKD	chronic kidney disease
CKD-MBD	CKD-mineral and bone disorder
CLL	chronic lymphocytic leukaemia
CML	chronic myeloid leukaemia
CNS	central nervous system
COMT	catechol-O-methyltransferase
COPD	chronic obstructive pulmonary disease
CPAP	continuous positive airway pressure
CRF	chronic renal failure
CSF	colony stimulating factor
CT	computed tomography
CVA	cerebrovascular accident
DCCT	Diabetes Control and Complications Trial
DPG	diphosphoglycerate
ECG	electrocardiogram
e.g.	exempli gratia (for example)
eGFR	estimated glomerular filtration rate
EGFR	epidermal growth factor receptor
EPS	extracellular polymeric substance
BFU-E	erythroid burst-forming unit
CFU-E	erythroid colony forming unit ,
ESR	erythrocyte sedimentation rate
ESV	end systolic volume
FAP	fluorapatite
FEV1	forced expiratory volume
FRC	functional residual capacity
FSH	follicle stimulating hormone
FVC	forced vital capacity
GA	general anaesthesia
GABA	gamma-aminobutyric acid
GORD	gastro-oesophageal reflux disease
GCF	gingival crevicular fluid
GHRH	growth hormone releasing hormone
GI	gastrointestinal
GLP-1	glucagon like peptide-1
GTN	glyceryl trinitrate
HAP	hydroxyapatite

HbA1c	glycated haemoglobin
HERS	Hertwig's epithelial root sheath
HIV	human immunodeficiency virus
HLA	human leukocyte antigen
HPA axis	hypothalamic–pituitary–adrenal
HPV	human papilloma virus
HSC	haematopoietic stem cell
HSP	human heat shock protein
HPV	human papilloma virus
HIF-1	hypoxia inducible factor-1
i.e.	id est (that is)
IEE	internal enamel epithelium
Ig	immunoglobin
IL-1	interleukin 1
INR	international normalized ratio
KD	Kawasaki disease
LDL	Lipids
L-DOPA	levodopa
LH	luteinizing hormone
MHC	major histocompatibility complex
MMPs	matrix metalloproteinases
MDMA	methylenedioxymethamphetamine
MRI	magnetic resonance imaging
MSC	mesenchymal stem cells
MI	myocardial infarction
MIP	maximal Intercuspal position
MOA	monoamine oxidase
MS	multiple sclerosis
MSA	multiple system atrophy
MNG	multinodular goitre
MROJ	medication-related osteonecrosis of the jaw
NK	natural killer
NICE	National Institute for Health and Care Excellence
NOAC	novel oral anticoagulant
NS	necrotizing sialometaplasia
NSAIDs	non-steroidal anti-inflammatory drugs
RANK	nuclear factor kappa-B
OSA	obstructive sleep apnoea
OPG	osteoprotegerin
PAF	platelet activating factor

PAMP	pathogen associated molecular pattern
PDL	periodontal ligament
PEP	post-exposure prophylaxis
PG	prostaglandins
PMN	polymorphonuclear leucocyte
PPE	personal protective equipment
PPI	proton pump inhibitor
PRR	pattern recognition receptor
PT	prothrombin time
PTC	papillary thyroid carcinoma
PTH	parathyroid hormone
PVS	Plummer–Vinson or Paterson–Brown–Kelly syndrome
RANKL	RANK ligand
RAS	recurrent aphthous stomatitis
RBC	red blood cell
RES	reticuloendothelial system
Rh	Rhesus
ROS	reactive oxygen species
SA	sinoatrial
SIRS	systemic inflammatory response syndrome
TBG	thyroxine-binding globulin
TRE	thyroid hormone response elements
TRH	thyrotrophin releasing hormone
TRPV1	transient receptor potential vanilloid receptor subtype 1
TSG	tumour suppressor gene
TSH	thyroid stimulating hormone
TSL	Tooth surface loss
TNF	tumor necrosis factor
vCJD	variant Creutzfeldt-Jakob Disease
WBC	white blood cell

Chapter 1

Oral cavity and gut

Tooth formation 2
Tooth eruption 8
Composition of dental hard tissues 12
Enamel 14
Dentine/pulp-dentine complex 15
Cementum 16
Periodontal tissues 18
Dental caries 22
Fluoride in caries prevention 26
Diet in caries prevention 28
The digestive tract 30
Diet and nutrition 34
Problems with diet and nutrition 36

Tooth formation

The early embryo starts as a ball of undifferentiated cells, then organizes into a 3-layered disc:

- Ectoderm—is the origin of skin and infolds to form the nervous system, sensory cells (of eyes, nose, etc), and dental enamel
- Mesoderm—is the origin of connective tissue, bone, muscle, kidneys, gonads, and spleen
- Endoderm—is the origin of epithelial lining of gut and respiratory systems, the parenchyma of liver and pancreas.

Some ectoderm cells that are involved in infolding to form the neural tube (and subsequently the central nervous system [CNS]) become specialized neural crest cells. These migrate throughout the embryo for specialized purposes and can differentiate into a wide range of cell types and tissues: neurons, glial cells, melanocytes, dermis, tendons, cartilage, bone, and dentine. It is thought that some neural crest derived cells retain some of this potential and may hold promise for regeneration of dental tissue in the adult.

The process of tooth formation starts at 5–6 weeks in utero with the formation of the dental lamina. This is a thickening of the ectoderm extending from the lining of the primitive oral cavity down into the underlying ectomesenchyme. Within this dental lamina, focal bud-like thickenings map out the sites of the future teeth, 20 for the primary dentition and later 32 for the permanent. These ectoderm buds together with a surrounding aggregation of ectomesenchymal cells form the earliest stage of the tooth germ. There are 6 stages in which the crown of the tooth is formed (➔ See Table 1.1). The process progresses from the cusp tip apically towards the root with the outer shape of the crown fully formed before root development starts. (➔ See Fig. 1.1 and 1.2)

The tooth germ comprises:

- *Enamel organ* develops into the enamel (ectodermal origin)
- *Dental papilla* develops into the dentine and pulp (neuro-ectodermal origin)
- *Dental follicle (sac)* develops into the periodontal ligament (neuro-ectodermal origin).

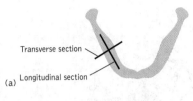

(a)

Longitudinal section

Tranverse section

Preodontogenesis

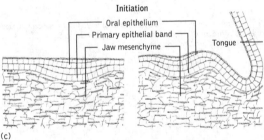

Oral epithelium
Jaw mesenchyme
Lingual
Mesial
Distal
Buccal
Tongue

(b)

Initiation

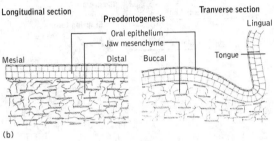

Oral epithelium
Primary epithelial band
Jaw mesenchyme
Tongue

(c)

Dental lamina

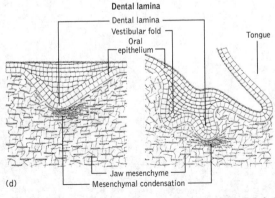

Dental lamina
Vestibular fold
Oral epithelium
Tongue

Jaw mesenchyme
Mesenchymal condensation

(d)

Fig. 1.1 Initiation stage of tooth development. Reproduced from Scully, C. *Oxford Handbook of Applied Dental Sciences* (2003), with permission from Oxford University Press.

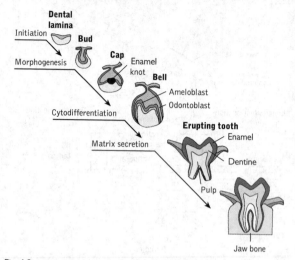

Fig. 1.2 Diagram showing developmental stages of teeth from initiation to eruption. Reproduced from Scully, C. *Oxford Handbook of Applied Dental Sciences* (2003), with permission from Oxford University Press.

Table 1.1 Stages of tooth development

Timing in utero	Stage	Activity	Potential problems
6 weeks	Initiation	Ectoderm of the primitive stomodeum thickens locally to form dental lamina which maps the later dental arch	Oligodontia (partial anodontia)
		Mesenchyme forms neural crest which migrates to the tooth germ	Supernumeraries
8 weeks	Bud	Each dental lamina develops 10 buds	Macro or microdontia
9–10 weeks	Cap	The enamel organ maps out the shape of the crown	
		Dental papilla is surrounded by follicle and sac	
11–12 weeks	Bell	Differentiation of 4 layers Stratum intermedium Inner enamel epithelium Outer dental papilla Central cells of dental papilla	
	Appositional	Dentine and enamel are laid down. Internal enamel epithelium (IEE) cells become preameloblasts which induce odontoblasts to produce predentine. The basement membrane disintegrates, allowing preodontoblasts and preameloblasts to come into contact. Predentine mineralizes and induces enamel matrix production from Tome's process of ameloblasts. Enamel matrix mineralizes very quickly (dentine facilitates nucleation). Odontoblast processes are left as the odontoblast cell bodies continue to lay down more dentine. Centres of calcification (calcospherites) fuse. At the odontoblast layer, there is always a layer of predentine throughout life. Stellate reticulum collapses and nutrients are then supplied from blood supply outside the outer enamel epithelium.	Enamel/dentine dysplasia

(Continued)

Table 1.1 (Contd.)

Timing in utero	Stage	Activity	Potential problems
	Enamel maturation	Mineral ion uptake increases and crystals grow wider and thicken. Water and organic content are removed from the enamel. At the end of this stage the enamel epithelium degenerates.	
	Root formation	Once the crown has formed, at the cervical loop, outer and inner enamel epithelium become adjacent (stellate reticulum and stellate intermedium having collapsed). These 2 layers form the Hertwig's epithelial root sheath (HERS) which induces dentine formation between dental papilla and follicle. When complete the basement membrane and HERS disintegrate and some cells remain in a mesh of strands and islands (rests of Malassez). Undifferentiated cells in the dental papilla contact the root dentine and become cementoblasts which secrete cementoid matrix which mineralizes to cementum. Fibroblasts are induced to form periodontal ligament. Hyaline layer of cementum is next to the root dentine, a 10 micron highly mineralized layer which allows the first attachment of periodontal ligament fibres. Acellular cementum is found near the cervical area. Cementoblasts become encased in their own cementum as cementocytes in cellular cement. Root formation takes around 1.5 years from eruption for primary teeth and 2–3 years for permanent teeth.	Enamel pearls (blob of enamel formed on the root by misplaced ameloblasts). Dilaceration— bend in the root due to trauma. Accessory roots Concrescence— teeth joined by cementum

Tooth eruption

Eruption brings the tooth from its developmental position into its functional position. The mechanism is not fully understood. The dental follicle is crucial (it later becomes the periodontal ligament). It seems the tooth is pushed rather than pulled—there does not seem to be a traction force. The dental follicle evolves to produce a complete crown then transforming growth hormone is released which attracts osteoclasts and macrophages which cause bone remodelling around the crown. Next, the overlying soft tissue breaks down releasing enamel matrix protein which may be part of teething—rhinitis, fever, and inflammation of soft tissue around the erupting crown. Growth and thyroid hormones moderate eruption. (➔ See Fig. 1.3 for example of developing premolars.)

The mechanisms of eruption are not fully understood but factors potentially contributing to eruption are as follows.

- Root formation
  - Root growth is often happening at the same time as active eruption but seems to follow eruption rather than cause it, e.g. rootless teeth will erupt, teeth with a closed apex can still erupt.
- Tissue fluid hydrostatic pressure
  - This mechanism is seen as highly likely. Minute changes in tooth position are synchronized to the pulse and there is a diurnal pattern to eruption across the day. Changes in tissue pressure have been recorded corresponding to eruption activity, increased vascularity, and fenestrations in vasculature producing a swollen ground substance.

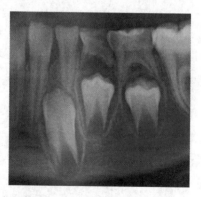

Fig. 1.3 Developing permanent canine and premolars.
Note: crown is fully formed and root formation is underway.

- Bone remodelling
  - Bone is certainly remodelled during tooth eruption (e.g. resorption locally to accommodate the developing clinical crown) but it seems not to be a major motive force.
- Periodontal ligament
  - Fibroblasts migrate along the periodontal ligament at the same rate as teeth erupt but this is thought to be a passive process and there seems to be no traction force here.

Problems of delayed eruption

Tooth eruption dates vary from person to person and up to 1 year either side of the given dates should be allowed (➔ See Table 1.2 and 1.3). Exfoliation of primary teeth and eruption of any teeth would normally be symmetrical so any 1-sided delay, beyond a few months, should be investigated. Causes for delay are most commonly local obstruction by a supernumerary or impacted tooth or because there is insufficient space for it to erupt into. Rarely systemic conditions are the cause, e.g.

- Hypothyroid—reduced levels of thyroid hormone
- Gardner's syndrome—polyposis coli and multiple jaw cysts
- Down's syndrome—learning disability, immune and cardiovascular defects
- Cleidocranial dysostosis—bone defects, unerupted supernumaries, dentigerous cysts
- Rickets—vitamin D deficiency during bone development
- Hereditary gingival fibromatosis—excess gingival tissue
- Cherubism—giant cell lesions in mandible+/- maxilla.

Even after the tooth is fully erupted there continues to be an adaptive process of remodelling bone and cementum which maintains the teeth in occlusal contact and vertical dimension. Forces on teeth, whether continuous or intermittent, during eruption can slow, stop or reverse eruption or redirect its path.

Summary of chronology of tooth development

➔ See Fig. 1.4 for primary teeth and Fig. 1.5 for permanent teeth.

Crown completion
Primary crown is complete:
Eruption date × 0.5 approximately

Permanent crown is complete:

6 1 2 3	3 years before eruption
3 4 5 7 8	5 years before eruption

Root completion

Primary	1–1.5 years after eruption
Permanent	2–3 years after eruption

Total development time

Primary	2–4 years
Permanent	12 years

Root resorption of primary teeth commences almost as soon as formation is complete. Exfoliation usually occurs several months before eruption of permanent successor.

Table 1.2 Eruption dates for permanent teeth

	Starts calcifying	Crown completed	Eruption
Upper 1	3–4 months		7–8 years
Lower 1		4–5 years	6–7 years
Upper 2	10–12 months		8–9 years
Lower 2	3–4 months		7–8 years
Upper 3	4–5 months	6–7 years	11–12 years
Lower 3			9–10 years
Upper 4	1.5–2 years	5–6 years	10–12 years
Lower 4			
Upper 5	2–2.5 years	6–7 years	10–12 years
Lower 5			
Upper & lower 6	Birth or just before	2.5–3 years	6–7 years
Upper & lower 7	2.5–3 years	7–8 years	12–13 years
Upper & lower 8	7–10 years Earlier for uppers, later for lowers	12–16 years	17–21 years

van Beek GC (1983) Dental Morphology: An Illustrated Guide. Wright.

Table 1.3 Eruption dates for primary teeth

	Starts calcifying	Crown completed	Eruption
Upper A	3–4.5 months in utero	4–5 months	7.5 months
Lower A			6.5 months
Upper B			8 months
Lower B			7 months
Upper C	5 months in utero	9 months	16–20 months
Lower C			
Upper D	5 months in utero	6 months	12–16 months
Lower D			
Upper E	6 months in utero	10–12 months	20–30 months
Lower E			

van Beek GC (1983) Dental Morphology: An Illustrated Guide. Wright.

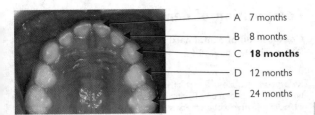

A   7 months
B   8 months
C   **18 months**
D   12 months
E   24 months

Fig. 1.4 Eruption of primary teeth.

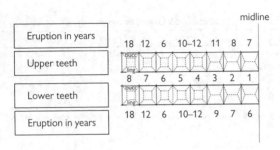

midline

Eruption in years	18	12	6	10–12	11	8	7
Upper teeth							
	8	7	6	5	4	3	2	1
Lower teeth							
Eruption in years	18	12	6	10–12	9	7	6

Fig. 1.5 Eruption of permanent teeth.

Composition of dental hard tissues

Composition of dental hard tissues
➔ See Table 1.4 and Fig. 1.6.

Resorption
Resorption of bone is a part of normal maintenance and tooth resorption is key to exfoliation of primary teeth. The process of activation and inhibition of osteoclastic activity is finely adjusted and at a histological level root resorption is common. Osteoclasts are responsible for resorption of bone, teeth, and cartilage. Osteoclasts are large multinucleate cells which lie in lacunae (Howship's) or crypts on hard tissue surfaces. Their prominent

Table 1.4 Composition of dental hard tissues by weight

	Inorganic	Organic	Water
Enamel	96%	1%	3%
Dentine	70%	20%	10%
Cementum	65%	23%	12%
Bone	60%	25%	15%

Berkovitz BKB, Holland GR, Moxham BJ. Oral Anatomy, Histology and Embryology 2009 Mosby.

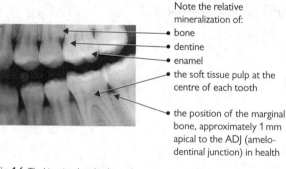

Note the relative mineralization of:
- bone
- dentine
- enamel
- the soft tissue pulp at the centre of each tooth
- the position of the marginal bone, approximately 1 mm apical to the ADJ (amelo-dentinal junction) in health

Fig. 1.6 The bitewing dental radiograph.

pseudopodia enable motility. Intracellular vesicles release acid and proteo-lytic enzymes into a resorptive compartment between cell and tissue surface which is carefully sealed from surrounding tissue. Chemical mediators (including tumour necrosis factor (TNF) cytokines) trigger macrophages and mononuclear cells to fuse and become osteoclasts. (⊙ See Fig. 1.7 for example of severe resorption.)

Factors promoting resorption
- Cytokines released during tissue damage
- Parathyroid hormone in response to low serum calcium
- Bacterial lipopolysaccharides.

Factors inhibiting resorption
- Osteoprotegerin (osteoclast inhibitory factor) released by stromal cells and osteoblasts.

Clinical application
Manifestations of resorption include:
- Exfoliation of primary teeth is achieved by resorption of the primary tooth roots as a normal part of dental development
- Responses to tissue injury
- Teeth can respond in a number of ways when subjected to trauma:
  - External surface resorption (often self-limiting)
  - External inflammatory root resorption
  - External replacement resorption (ankylosis)
  - External cervical resorption
  - Internal resorption can take similar forms but originates from pulpal inflammation.

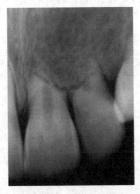

Fig. 1.7 Severe external root resorption.

Enamel

Derives from the enamel organ.

Enamel is a unique hard tissue, the hardest and most highly mineralized tissue of the human body. Enamel is acellular and non-vital and so cannot repair itself. However, enamel is permeable to water and small molecules and is in dynamic chemical equilibrium with the oral environment.

Enamel prisms

The enamel prism is the basic unit that makes up the enamel. The width of a prism is about 5 μm at the ADJ but widens towards the enamel surface. Along the length of the prism are cross-striations at 4 μm intervals, marking daily rest phases during enamel formation and a change in crystallite orientation. These prisms are, in turn, made up of crystallites, which are much smaller hexagonal rods. These crystallites are formed by specialized cells, ameloblasts, and pass from near to the ADJ out towards the tooth surface in a roughly perpendicular direction. Individual prisms follow a gently tortuous, undulating course, especially in the cuspal area.

On cross-section prisms show a 'keyhole' appearance, with a 'head' and 'tail' portion. Between prisms is the interprismatic region where there is a sharp change in crystallite direction and an increased water and organic content. Within the head portion of the prisms, crystallites are tightly packed with their long axes perfectly aligned with the long axis of the enamel prism. In the tail part of the prism, crystallite orientation is considered less well organized and there is a greater water and organic matrix content. Both inter-prismatic and tail portion of the prism are thought to serve a 'shock-absorbing' function.

Incisal edges and cusps tips

Prisms in the cuspal and incisal regions follow a rather complicated spiralling course which is thought to allow the brittle enamel to better withstand occlusal forces.

Surface enamel

This is the last part of the enamel prism to form. The surface tends to be harder and less soluble than the subsurface enamel due to higher levels of fluoride. In primary teeth and most permanent teeth the surface layer (for 30 μm) has no prism structure and so is termed aprismatic.

Striae of Retzius

These are incremental lines. It is thought that they mark rest periods during enamel formation and a change in crystallite orientation. In cross-section they look like concentric rings, like the growth rings of a tree. In longitudinal sections, they run obliquely upwards and outward towards the enamel surface. On erupted teeth, they may be seen to reach the surface as perikymata (fine horizontal lines running across the surface of the tooth).

The neo-natal line is an exaggerated incremental line found in teeth which began to form before birth (i.e. primary teeth and first permanent molars) and corresponds to the physiological and metabolic upheaval of birth.

The **amelo-dentinal junction** is the region of the tooth where the enamel and dentine first began to form. The junction is not straight but comprises dome-shaped protuberances of the under surface of the enamel fitting into depressions in the dentine surface (so it has a scalloped appearance in sections).

Dentine/pulp-dentine complex

Derives from the dental papilla.

Dentine and pulp function closely together. Dentine derives from the dental papilla from neural crest cells and pulp derives from the residual central core of the dental papilla. Odontoblasts form the dentine and retreat towards the centre of the tooth as the dentine is progressively laid down. As they retreat they leave a projection of the cell body, the odontoblast process, within tubules encased in the dentine. The dentine tubules may also contain afferent nerve terminals and processes of some immunocompetent cells. Dentinal tubules also contain dentinal fluid which is derived from extracellular fluid in the pulp. Hence, if the pulp is damaged or removed the dentine becomes drier and the colour of the tooth may darken. The pulp supplies nutrients and innervation to the dentine. The nerve fibres are mainly afferent but include sympathetic supply to blood vessels too. They range from myelinated large, medium and small and non-myelinated. Afferent fibres form a plexus, (the plexus of Raschow) under the odontoblasts and unmyelinated branches pass from it towards the odontoblasts and dentine. Essentially the only sensation that normally arises from the pulp is pain. This is regardless of the stimulus, e.g. heat or cold applied to the intact tooth, drying of an exposed dentine surface, trauma to dentine or pulp.

Dentine is of several types:

- Mantle dentine—initial innermost layer formed closest to the ADJ is least mineralized layer
- Primary dentine—the primary shape of the mature dentine
- Secondary dentine—formed after root formation is complete and slowly formed with ageing
- Tertiary dentine—formed in response to trauma and is of 2 types:
  - **Reactionary tertiary dentine** is laid down by the original odontoblasts.
  - **Reparative tertiary dentine** occurs where the original odontoblasts in that area have been destroyed and newly differentiated odontoblasts have taken on the role.

Cementum

Derives from the dental follicle.

Covers the root surface and is formed throughout life. Cementoblasts produce intrinsic collagen fibres and deposit cementum organic matrix (proteoglycans, glycoproteins, and phosphoproteins) into lamellar layers. Fibres from periodontal ligaments (also known as Sharpey's fibres) attach to or fuse with cementum intrinsic collagen. Cementum deposition continues throughout life in a rhythmic process shown in incremental lines. Cementum is thickest in the apical third and in the furcation areas. It is also thicker in distal surfaces than in mesial surfaces, probably because of functional stimulation from mesial drift over time. Previous layers of cementum help initiate mineralization of newer layers. The last formed non-mineralized layer is precementum. This allows periodontal ligament fibres to attach and adjust to varying functions. Cementum is less readily resorbed than bone and protects the dentine but there is ongoing resorption and repair in the cementum and dentine of most permanent teeth.

- Acellular cementum forms first and covers the cervical 2/3 of the root. It is formed slowly and is well mineralized. Fibres from the periodontal ligament insert into it and are known as Sharpey fibres.
- Cellular cementum forms at the apex and furcation. It forms more rapidly and some cementoblasts become trapped within the cementum (seen as cementocytes in lacunae) with numerous interconnecting extensions in the form of a 'spider web'.
- Intermediate cementum—an afibrillar and acellular layer, 10–20 μm thick, between dentine and cementum. This is formed by the HERS which then fragments thus triggering dental follicle cells to differentiate into cementoblasts and initiate cementum deposition.

Commonly (in 60%) the cementum overlaps the enamel and there is a butt joint in around 30%. In 10% there is a gap with no cementum, exposing dentine and sensitivity may arise. Cementum becomes exposed to the oral environment where loss of attachment occurs. It is prone to caries and becomes permeated by organic and inorganic substances to which it is exposed as well as oral bacteria.

Hypercementosis (excessive cementum)

May be associated with:
- Functional stress, e.g. bruxism, teeth clenching, occlusal trauma
- Periapical inflammation, e.g. granuloma
- But in many cases there is no obvious associated factor.

Hypercementosis can complicate tooth extraction.

Periodontal tissues

Derives from the dental follicle.
  Periodontal ligament derives from the dental follicle
  Functions:
1. Tooth support
2. Contribution to eruption
3. Bone and cementum formation
4. Mechano-receptors for mastication

The support for the teeth is provided by fibres, vascular pressure, and ground substance. The blood supply is rich mainly coming from vessels from the bone and gingivae. There is a plexus of capillary loops in the crevicular area. Vessels have lots of fenestrations.
  The fibre content is composed of:
• Collagen
• Elastin associated with blood vessels
• Oxytalan, a possible precursor of elastin.

The collagen fibres are bundled together in principal fibres 5 μm across. They run in various directions:
1. Interdental/alveolar crest
2. Horizontal
3. Oblique
4. Apical
5. Inter-radicular

Where principal fibres are embedded in bone or cementum, they are referred to as Sharpey's fibres. (➔ See Figs 1.8 and 1.9.)

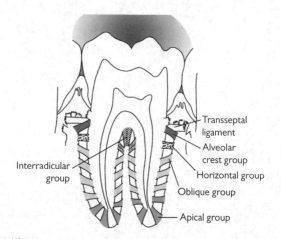

Interradicular group

Transseptal ligament

Alveolar crest group

Horizontal group

Oblique group

Apical group

Fig. 1.8 The 5 principal periodontal fibre groups. Reproduced from Scully, C. *Oxford Handbook of Applied Dental Sciences* (2003), with permission from Oxford University Press.

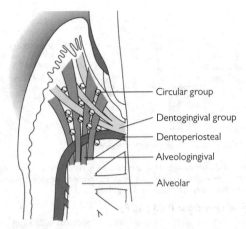

Fig. 1.9 The 5 gingival fibre groups. Reproduced from Scully, C. *Oxford Handbook of Applied Dental Sciences* (2003), with permission from Oxford University Press.

The cell content of the periodontal ligament is composed of:
• Connective tissue—fibroblasts, osteoblasts, cementoblasts
• Epithelium—rests of Malassez
• Immune cells—macrophages and mast cells
• Neurovascular cells.

The epithelial rests are concentrated at the periapical and cervical areas and if stimulated give rise to periapical or lateral periapical cysts.

Mechano-receptors are mainly Ruffini-type, slowly adapting stretch receptors, which relay signals via A-beta fibres of the trigeminal nerve to the trigeminal ganglion or mesencephalic nucleus of V. Two reflexes are triggered:
• Jaw opening reflex
• Masticatory–salivary reflex. This will stimulate saliva flow in response to gum chewing.

Crevicular epithelium
The gingival sulcus is lined by non-keratinized crevicular epithelium with very infolded interface with underlying connective tissue.

Junctional epithelium
The epithelial attachment is a non-keratinized high turnover epithelium composed of cells that uniquely have two basal laminae—one adjacent to lamina propria (underlying vascular connective tissue) and the other adjacent to enamel/dentine/cementum. There are large intercellular spaces

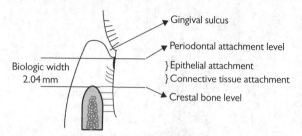

Fig. 1.10 Biologic width as reported by Gargiulo et al[1].

with fewer desmosomes. This feature allows crevicular fluid and defence cells into the gingival crevice. The gingiva also contain dense collagen fibre bundles which keep the tissue firm (Fig. 1.9).

Gingival crevicular fluid (GCF)

Derived from plasma it emerges from the junctional epithelium into the gingival crevice. Flow is greatly increased in inflammation and allows cellular and humoral components of blood to reach the tooth surface. It is also high in Ca^{2+} and phosphates.

Biologic width is the dimension of the soft tissue, which is attached to the portion of the tooth coronal to the crest of the alveolar bone. Restorative margins which encroach on this area often result in gingival inflammation, loss of clinical attachment and bone loss, due to plaque accumulation. There is a general agreement to aim for around 3 mm between the restorative margin and the alveolar bone crest (2 mm of biologic width and 1 mm for the gingival sulcus) and that encroachment on the gingival sulcus should be kept to a minimum. This is based on the finding of 2.04 mm as the mean biologic width in the work of Gargiulo et al[1], although there is variation around this. (➜ See Fig. 1.10.)

Reference

[1] Gargiulo, AW, Wentz, F & Orban, B. (1961) Dimensions and relations of the dentogingival junction in humans. *J Periodontol* **32**: 261–267.

Dental caries

The carious process is the dynamic demineralizing and remineralizing processes resulting from microbial metabolism on the tooth surface. Over time it may result in a net loss of mineral, and subsequently cavitation[2]. The ethical, logical approach to managing caries in an individual patient is to assess the level of risk and help the patient reduce their level of risk and to detect any lesions early and work with the patient to remineralize them. Increasingly this is what patients expect of the profession.

Epidemiology

It is one of the most common diseases and the most common cause of tooth loss at all ages in the UK. As defined above, it is a ubiquitous process, wherever sugar is consumed by dentate people. Dental surveys only include obvious dentine caries. They do this in order to limit the amount of variability between surveys (the larger the lesion the less disagreement between examiners) so surveys only show part of the problem for every detected lesion, there will be many others at earlier stage of demineralization and lesions in inaccessible areas. This is the so called 'iceberg' of dental caries. As with an iceberg, most of the bulk of it is unseen, as it were, beneath the water line.

Aetiology

The fundamental pathology is based on the occurrence of 4 factors together:
- Free sugars
- Bacterial activity producing acid
- Susceptible tooth surface—especially stagnation areas
- Time of exposure—worst if prolonged and frequent exposure to free sugars.

Because plaque formation is unavoidable, it is clear that the presence of free sugars is the primary determinant. However, many biological, socio-economic, and behavioural interacting factors will affect the outcomes.

Risk factors and markers

Biological
- Inadequate salivary flow
- Composition of saliva
- Cariogenic oral flora
- Insufficient fluoride exposure
- Gingival recession exposing vulnerable root dentine
- Immunological and genetic factors.

Socio-economic and behavioural
- Living in deprivation
- Inadequate oral hygiene
- Plaque retentive factors, e.g. denture, orthodontic appliance
- Caries in primary caregiver or family.

Free sugars

There is overwhelming evidence for the essential role of free sugars in the aetiology of dental caries. The term 'free sugars' comprises all monosaccharides and disaccharides added to foods by the manufacturer, cook or consumer, plus sugars naturally present in honey, syrups, and unsweetened fruit juices. Under this definition lactose, when naturally present in milk and milk products, and sugars contained within the cellular structure of foods, are excluded. Sucrose is considered the most cariogenic sugar. It is used by plaque bacteria in anaerobic fermentation to produce acid (lactic, acetic, propionic) and also contributes to the synthesis of extracellular polysaccharides.

Bacterial activity

The mouth contains a complex eco-system of hundreds of types of bacteria. Dental plaque is the complex community of micro-organisms embedded in a matrix of polymers (which originates from both bacteria and saliva). Plaque forms continually on any hard surfaces in the mouth (including dentures) but most readily in areas of stagnation, e.g. interproximally, along the gingival margin and in pits, fissures, and any deficiencies in the surface. It is an example of a biofilm, i.e. a community of micro-organisms attached to a surface. The plaque comprises: extracellular polymeric substance (EPS) matrix, bacteria (alive and dead), host debris, and yeasts. Towards the deeper layers of plaque, there is a gradient, with reducing nutrients, oxygen, and pH. The flora varies through these layers with a potential for complex interactions among organisms, e.g. exchange of genes and quorum sensing.

The first stage in plaque formation is the acquired pellicle, formed by the tooth surface absorbing salivary proteins and glycoproteins, plus some bacterial molecules. This remains undisturbed by tooth brushing and is only removed by prophylaxis by rotary brush or rubber cup. The acquired pellicle attracts some microbes loosely and others bind strongly via adhesins in the cell wall interacting with receptors in the acquired pellicle. Late colonizers may then attach to the early colonizers (coaggregation). The cells then continue to divide and produce a complex interacting microbial community.

In the past specific acidogenic species of bacteria, e.g. *Streptococcus mutans*, were named as the main causative agent. But more recent understanding is that multiple microorganisms are thought to act collectively, probably synergistically, in the initiation and progression of the lesion. Among these are:

- Lactobacilli—in dentine caries, root caries, rampant caries
- *Actinomyces naeslundii*—in dentine and root caries
- Gram-positives e.g. (*A. naeslundii*, *A. odontolyticus*, *Propionibacterium* spp., *Eubacterium* spp.) in deep lesions
- Gram-negatives (e.g. *Fusobacterium* spp., *Capnocytophaga* spp., *Veillonella* spp.) in deep lesions.

Complex interaction occur between them, e.g. *Veillonella* metabolizes lactic acid to less cariogenic acetic and propionic acids.

Progression of caries

Enamel caries is seen as a white area at locations of plaque stagnation and is primarily a chemical process driven by the presence of dental plaque at the surface. There is an advancing front of demineralization releasing mineral that diffuses towards the surface. Near the surface it tends to redeposit under the influence of higher fluoride levels in surface enamel and plaque and supersaturated calcium and phosphate in saliva and plaque fluid. If the conditions persist then eventually the surface layer will become demineralized, increasingly fragile, and eventually breakdown.

Dentine caries is initiated at around the same time as the surface breaks down and a cavity forms. This allows bacteria to invade the tissue, especially the dentinal tubules. In addition to continuing demineralization, the bacteria can produce proteolytic enzymes which break down the organic matrix. In dentine caries 2 layers are observable.

- Infected carious dentine, the outermost layer, not capable of remineralizing, nonvital, insensitive
- Affected carious dentine, an inner layer, is capable of remineralizing, vital, sensitive

In cavity preparation, the outer, infected carious dentine is entirely removed but the inner carious dentine may be retained.

Root caries is especially hazardous.
- The critical pH for dentine demineralization is higher than enamel at around 6.3.
- The preventive effect of fluoride is less effective against dentine caries and fluoride concentrations need to be higher for an equivalent effect.
- Root caries can be difficult to detect, commonly approximally, and at restoration margins.

Reference

[2] Fejerskov, O. (1997) Concepts of dental caries and their consequences for understanding the disease. *Community Dent Oral Epidemiol* **25**: 5–12.

Fluoride in caries prevention

Fluoride action in caries prevention

The main anti-caries action of fluoride is as a catalyst in both promoting remineralization and inhibiting demineralization. The dental calcified tissues are mainly hydroxyapatite (HAP) (Ca_{10} $(PO_4)_6$ $(OH)_2$) but several other ions are incorporated into the HAP lattice. Incorporation of hydrogen phosphate, carbonate, and magnesium ions makes the structure more unstable and soluble. Fluoride ions can substitute for OH groups in the crystal lattice and stabilize the apatite structure, reducing the critical pH to 4.7. However, in the superficial layers of enamel, less than 5% of the OH groups of HAP are replaced by fluoride and thus fluorapatite (FAP) has very little effect on caries susceptibility and solubility of HAP.

When fluoride products are applied to teeth, a protective layer of calcium fluoride is formed (CaF_2). In acid conditions, CaF_2 releases F ions and in the supersaturated solution resulting, FAP is laid down preferentially as the pH returns to resting levels. Fluoride ions are also adsorbed onto crystals giving direct protection. Early enamel lesions are more porous and fluoride ions are concentrated in here. Hence, healing early lesions are then less susceptible to caries progression.

Excess fluoride

Acute overdose

May occur if excess is ingested from dental products. This is most likely to occur in children. The toxic dose of 5 mg/kg means that a quarter of a 100 g tube of family toothpaste ingested by a 1-year-old child may potentially be lethal. Symptoms include: nausea, vomiting, epigastric pain, respiratory and cardiac depression, and convulsions, and a coma may follow. Immediate management is to induce vomiting and administer a calcium solution, e.g. milk, to help bind any remaining free fluoride in the gut. Urgent hospital admission is required.

Chronic systemic exposure to excess fluoride

Gives rise to systemic fluorosis characterized by excess calcification of bone, bony exostoses, stiff and painful joints especially in the spine. This can occur at total fluoride intakes above about 6 mg/day. High water fluoride levels are endemic in many parts of the world, depending on the geology of the rock with which the water has been in contact and de-fluoridation of the supply is necessary as a public health measure in such areas.

Mild excess of fluoride

The ameloblast is the most sensitive to excess fluoride. At low levels during the secretory phase of enamel formation then hypercalcification will occur. If calcification has started then hypocalcification will result. During the maturation phase, there is failure to increase mineral content and failure to remove protein and water. The resulting enamel is more porous than normal. In mild cases, this results in surface effects such as fine white lines along the perikymata or diffuse white opacities which can be removed with wear or microabrasion. In more severe cases, defects may include the whole thickness of enamel and porosities pick up staining in the mouth, hence appearing brown. Pitting may also occur and restorative techniques such as direct resin composites and veneers will be needed to mask the defects.

Preventing excess fluoride ingestion

Using fluoride in caries prevention requires a balancing of potential risks and benefits. The anti-caries effect increases with dosage of fluoride, as does the risk of dental fluorosis in children. Dental fluorosis is only a risk during enamel formation and usually it is only an aesthetic problem. Hence, the risk of dental fluorosis is of aesthetic concern but is dramatically reduced once the crowns of permanent incisors, canines, and premolars are complete around the age of 7 years. Other advice to limit the risk of dental fluorosis in children is:

• Keep toothpaste out of reach of children
• Supervise children toothbrushing until at least the age of 7 years
• Use only a smear of toothpaste, pea sized amount from the age of 3 years
• Encourage children to spit out excess toothpaste.

Fluoride metabolism

Fluoride is absorbed from stomach and small intestine as hydrogen fluoride. It is taken up into calcified tissue, teeth (during their development), and remodelling bone. Excess fluoride is excreted in urine, freely filtered across glomerular capillaries, and reabsorbed to varying degrees depending on the pH, and so affected by diet, drugs, and metabolic disorders. The remainder is excreted in urine. Some 10–25% is not absorbed from the gut and passes through into faeces.

Diet in caries prevention

Plaque bacteria form organic acids (mainly lactic, also propionic and acetic) from sugars. These acids demineralize the dental hard tissue once the critical pH is reached. The pH returns to resting value, typically over 30–60 minutes and a period of remineralization occurs. The speed with which the resting pH level is achieved depends on several factors:
1. Salivary flow and composition
2. Other food/drinks consumed—sugar content, consistency, and time retained in the mouth

The Stephan curve (Fig. 1.11) gives a graphical representation of the effect of frequency of sugar consumption on demineralization.

The critical pH illustrated is that for enamel, pH5.5, but for dentine is higher at around 6.3, i.e. dentine demineralizes more readily in acid conditions. This critical pH varies with the calcium, phosphate, and fluoride saturation of the oral environment—saliva and plaque fluid. So acid drinks that contain calcium have a reduced erosive potential because the 'critical' pH value is reduced.

Salivary flow and composition

Buffering refers to an ability to resist changes in pH. In saliva and dental plaque fluid, this is achieved by excess H^+ being bound by bicarbonate, phosphate, or some proteins. Stimulating a high flow of saliva increases bicarbonate levels, increasing buffering, and directly raises the plaque pH. This is partly due to the high bicarbonate content and increased nitrogenous substrates, which are metabolized by bacteria to less acidic end products. This stimulated flow can be achieved by chewing gum. Cheese has similar action and also provides increased plaque concentrations of calcium and phosphate for remineralization.

Dietary change

The WHO (2015)[3] states that intake of free sugars at the level of 10% of total energy intake is associated with high caries rates for both adults and children even where fluoride is present in drinking water and toothpastes. Hence, WHO strongly recommends reducing the intake of free sugars to

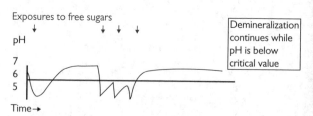

Fig. 1.11 Stephan curve.

less than 10% of total energy intake. Even below 5% there is a positive log-linear relationship between free sugar intake and caries experience. A further reduction of the intake to below 5% of total energy intake has been suggested and would have even greater benefit to caries reduction (PHE, 2015)[4]. Further benefits of dietary free sugar reduction include reduced risk of type 2 diabetes and of weight gain. The dental health priority is to reduce the frequency of sugar intake, even if the overall amount is unaltered, as a way of limiting demineralization.

Behaviour change

Most of our habitual behaviour is automatic, unthinking, and quite resistant to change so helping patients to change is difficult! An evidence-based approach is needed and elements of successful behaviour change might include (NICE, 2014)[5]:

- Help the patient understand the consequences of their behaviour and the benefits of change
- Encourage the patient to make a commitment to change
- Record the decision and set goals
- Do not attempt too much—plan easy steps
- Plan for coping with difficult situations where relapse is likely
- Encourage the patient to share their goals with others
- Continue to monitor and support the patient for at least a year.

Efforts to change behaviour at an individual level must acknowledge the powerful impact of the environment (family, peers, work, economic, political) and will be more likely to be effective if policy and interventions at community and wider population levels exist too[5]. Examples include: tax and pricing policy for sugar containing foods and drinks; controls on advertising (especially to children); health promotion in community settings—early years, schools, workplaces, hospitals, social care.

References

[3] WHO (2015) Guideline. Sugars intake for adults and children.
[4] PHE (Public Health England) (2015) SACN. Carbohydrates and health.
[5] NICE (2014) Behaviour change: individual approaches: Public health guideline [PH49].

The digestive tract

Progression along the gut

1. Oesophagus is a muscular tube leading to the stomach and usually closed off from the pharynx by the upper oesophageal sphincter which relaxes momentarily to allow the bolus to pass through at the end of the pharyngeal phase of swallowing. Ingested food progresses down the oesophagus aided by peristalsis. This is a co-ordinated wave of contraction behind the bolus and relaxation in front. This propels the bolus (even against gravity if necessary) towards the lower oesophageal sphincter.

2. Stomach acts as a reservoir and mixing chamber which churns the food and secretions into chyme and releases it in small amounts through the pyloric sphincter into the duodenum, while the bulk is kept in the stomach and subject to further churn. Gastric motility is reduced by sympathetic stimulation, e.g. following heavy exercise or blood loss. Gastric motility is increased by parasympathetic stimulation, mechanical distension, and release of gastrin (from G cells in gastric mucosa). Fat and acid in the duodenum slows gastric emptying, allowing time for neutralizing acid and absorbing lipids. This effect may be mediated by cholecystokinin and secretin by the small intestine in response to chyme.

3. Small intestine is the main site of digestion and absorption, offering an area said to be the size of a tennis pitch. It is about 4 m long and its cells are highly active, undergoing replacement every 6 days. The chyme which passes into the duodenum is acid and hypertonic. It is rapidly neutralized by bicarbonate, bile, and various enzymes. It also equilibrates and becomes isotonic. There are 3 discrete areas of small intestine:
   • Duodenum
   • Jejunum
   • Ileum.

The surface area of the small intestine is hugely increased by finger-like projections into the lumen (villi) each with a capillary network and central blind-ended lymphatic vessel (lacteal). The venous capillaries empty into the hepatic portal vein and the lacteals empty into the left subclavian vein via the thoracic duct. Between the villi are crypts the cells of which secrete up to 3 L/day of hypotonic fluid. Small intestine has 3 movements:
   • Segmentation—local phased spontaneous activity
   • Peristalsis—the main propulsion
   • Migratory motor complexes—several hours after a meal stronger propulsion sweeps the remnants towards the ileocaecal sphincter which opens in response to distension of the terminal ileum and distension of the caecum triggers it to close.

4. Large intestine is the main site for water and electrolyte absorption. There are 7 discrete areas of the large intestine: caecum; colon (ascending, transverse and descending) sigmoid colon, rectum, and the anal canal.

The large intestine abounds in bacteria, mostly anaerobic. These bacteria serve many useful purposes including: producing B_{12}, thiamine, riboflavin, breaking down cholesterol, some drugs, and food additives, bilirubin (converting it to non-pigmented metabolites), and the conversion of primary bile acids to secondary bile acids. Bacterial fermentation produces gas. Fatty acids produced by bacterial action here are thought to be protective against cancer and research continues to investigate the large intestine microflora. The large intestine has 2 movements:

- Segmentation—local phased spontaneous activity
- Mass movements 3–4 times daily—synchronized sustained contractions triggered by a meal (gastro-colic reflex) and perhaps involving gastrin.

The rectum has stretch receptors which stimulate parasympathetic activity via the sacral spinal cord producing contraction of the colon and releasing the internal anal sphincter. The rectum has two sphincters: internal anal sphincter supplied by parasympathetic system and external anal sphincter supplied by somatic motor supply and under conscious control.

Secretions

Gastric secretions

- Pepsins are released in an inactive form (pepsinogens) from the chief cells of the stomach wall and are spontaneously activated by the acid environment.
- HCl is produced by parietal cells. About 2 L per day are produced. Intracellular H^+ is exchanged for extracellular K^+ and a pH of 1.5–3.5 is achieved.
- Alkaline mucous (a viscous glycoprotein) is produced by mucous cells to protect the mucosa from being digested by pepsin or damaged by acid. Further protection is afforded by local mediators which respond to any mucosal irritation by thickening the mucous layer and stimulating bicarbonate production.
- Intrinsic factor is released—essential for later absorption of vitamin B^{12}.

Pancreatic secretions

About 1 L is produced each day by the pancreas, stimulated by cholecystokinin (CCK) which is triggered by the presence of chyme in the duodenum. Constituents include:

- Amylase which splits carbohydrate to monosaccharides
- Lipase which splits fats to fatty acids and glycerol
- RNAase /DNAase which spilt nucleic acids
- Proteolytic enzymes which split proteins to peptides and amino acids
- Water and bicarbonates which neutralize chyme.

Bile

- About 1 litre per day is produced by the liver. Bile is stored in the gall bladder and its release is triggered by CCK (and vagal stimulation) which causes contraction of gall bladder muscles and opening of the sphincter of Oddi which allows its release into the duodenum.
- Bile is formed, stimulated by gastrin, secretin, glucagon, and bile salts. There are 3 stages to bile production:
  - Formation of bile acid dependent fraction, a plasma-like fluid with bile salts, bile pigments, cholesterol, lecithin, and mucous. This passes to the bile ducts.

Table 1.5 Co-ordinating mechanisms in the gut

Secretin formed by the epithelial cells of the duodenum under the stimulus of acid contents from the stomach, released in blood	Stimulates pepsin release by from chief cells of stomach Inhibits gastric emptying Stimulates secretion of copious secretin of high HCO_3 pancreatic juice
Cholecystokinin (CCK) polypeptide hormone secreted from I cells of duodenum/upper jejunum stimulated by products of protein & fat digestion released into blood	Stimulates pepsin release by from chief cells of stomach Inhibits gastric emptying Stimulates gall bladder contraction, sphincter of Oddi relaxes and secretion of pancreatic enzymes
Mechanoreceptors detect stretch/stomach distension	Inhibits gastric emptying
Gastrin polypeptide hormone secreted by G cells of the pyloric glands	Strongly stimulates secretion of gastric acid and pepsin, and weakly stimulates secretion of pancreatic enzymes and gall bladder contraction
Vagal stimulation	Secretion of pancreatic enzymes Weak contraction of gall bladder

- Bile is modified by addition of water and bicarbonate (the bile acid independent fraction) as it passes along the bile duct.
- Bile is modified in the gall bladder which stores and concentrates bile while the sphincter of Oddi is closed (there is active Na transport out into the intercellular spaces and this draws water, Cl and HCO_3 with it).

Vomiting (emesis)

This is an elegant and complex reflex which protects the body from potential choking hazards and ingesting toxic materials. It allows the stomach contents to be ejected whilst the airway is protected and respiration temporarily suspended. Commonly vomiting occurs in 3 successive stages—nausea, retching, and vomiting. Vomiting is expulsion of gastric contents. It is usually accompanied by nausea, an unpleasant subjective experience linked with a desire to vomit. Retching is a strong involuntary effort to vomit but without expelling gastric contents. In retching the nasopharynx is closed, glottis is closed, upper oesophageal sphincter (mainly cricopharyngeus) is closed, the antrum of the stomach contracts and the fundus and cardia relax, and thoracic pressure is decreased and abdominal pressure is increased. This process may serve to position gastric contents and overcome oesophageal resistance in readiness for vomiting. The vomiting centre is not a discrete entity but a network of complexes in the medulla which trigger the sequence of events across respiratory, cardiovascular systems, and swallowing. Inputs are received from:

- Gastrointestinal (GI) tract—oropharynx, stomach, duodenum irritation
- Vestibular system—triggered in motion sickness

- Chemoreceptor trigger zone—triggered by
- Higher centres in the cortex and thalamus—mediating triggers of sight, smell, fear, memory

Activation involves motor, parasympathetic, and sympathetic nervous systems. Sympathetic activation leads to sweating, pallor, and increased heart rate. Parasympathetic activation leads to increased salivation at high flow. The striated duct cells do not have time for their usual reabsorption of HCO_3^- which gives the characteristic taste in the mouth before vomiting and contributes to increasing the pH prior to acidic stomach contents arriving in the mouth. There follows: contraction of abdominal muscles and diaphragm (increasing pressure in thorax and abdomen); lower oesophageal sphincter relaxes; deep inspiration is taken; nasopharynx and glottis are closed; intra-abdominal pressure rises and stomach contents are expelled.

Repeated vomiting may lead to dehydration and serious electrolyte and acid–base imbalance. Aspiration of vomit is a further hazard.

Clinical relevance

Retching is a common hazard during some dental procedures, especially impression taking, and some patients are particularly sensitive and easily provoked to retching. It is good to be forewarned by asking if they have undergone a certain procedure before and how it went. Precautions might include:

- A calm and empathic approach.
- Seating the impression posteriorly first so that excess runs forward rather than backward towards the pharynx.
- Positioning the patient. Opinion differ about this. A supine position allows the uvula to swing posteriorly away from the impression but any excess material will slump posteriorly too. An upright or hunched-forward position will allow excess to drain forwards but the uvula will swing forward and may be more likely to be stimulated.
- Ensuring a faster set by choice of material or increasing the temperature.
- Relaxing and distracting the patient, e.g. by focusing on breathing slowly through the nose or raising their legs. Presumably this strategy works by interference with input from higher centres.
- Habituation by gradually increasing challenge, e.g. applying toothbrush to hard palate progressively further palatally.
- Hypnosis, acupuncture, conscious sedation may be needed in severe cases.

Diet and nutrition

Appetite is complex and controlled by two centres in the hypothalamous, the satiety centre, and the hunger centre. Inputs that activate the satiety centre include: increasing blood glucose levels, gastric distension and leptin, a protein hormone, released by fat stores. There are also inputs from higher centres. The net response after eating is to inhibit the hunger centre. As this effect fades, appetite returns.

Dietary advice

Advice on healthy eating changes in line with research but currently includes consuming:

* Plenty of starchy foods such as potatoes, rice, bread, and pasta
* At least 5 portions of fruit and vegetables daily
* Some beans, pulses, fish, eggs, meat, and other protein
* Two portions of fish a week, one of which is oily
* Some dairy products or dairy alternatives, e.g. soya based
* Six to eight glasses (about 1.2 litres) of water, or other fluids, daily.

Foods and drinks high in fat, salt, and/or sugar should be taken only in small amounts, infrequently.

Protein

Dietary requirement is around 40–50 g/per day but intake is commonly twice this. A piece of meat the thickness and size of the palm is sufficient and there are vegetarian alternatives. If excess is eaten it is used for energy and yields 4 kcal/g. The component units of proteins are amino acids. Twenty amino acids are found in human and mammal cells of which 10 can be synthesized by the body but 10 cannot and so must be supplied in the diet. A varied diet is needed if all these essential amino acids are to be supplied.

Digestion is by pepsins (in the stomach) and peptidases from pancreatic secretion and in the brush border of villi.

Absorption is by carrier proteins in duodenum and jejunum.

Fat

Fats are the most energy dense of food components, yielding 9 kcal/g. Dietary recommendations are for fat to account for at most 35% of dietary energy. Fats are categorized as saturated (single bonded structure) or unsaturated (double bonds). It used to be thought that saturated fats, typically found in meat, were implicated in cardiovascular disease and raising blood cholesterol but this view has changed to focus on added sugar.

Digestion is complicated by the problem of fat not being water soluble.

Stomach churning and lipase emulsifies the mix, producing droplets of lipid. These are acted on by pancreatic lipase producing free fatty acids and monoglycerides.

Absorption is aided by these becoming incorporated into bile micelles and at the microvilli dissolves into the lipid cell membrane. Once within the cell the endoplasmic reticulum reassembles triglycerides which are transported by the Golgi apparatus to exit the cell into interstitial fluid and the lymphatics.

Carbohydrate

Carbohydrates have an energy yield of 4 kcal/g. Simple sugars are quickly absorbed and produce a spike of blood glucose. Complex carbohydrates are absorbed more slowly and allow a more controlled stable glucose level to be maintained. Some polysaccharides are not digested, e.g. cellulose and constitute dietary fibre which passes through unaltered to the faeces.

Digestion of starch starts with salivary amylase and continues with pancreatic amylase resulting in tri- and di- saccharides and dextrins.

Enzymes released from the brush border break down larger sugars to monosaccharides.

Absorption of carbohydrates takes place in the duodenum and jejunum. Monosaccharides from the lumen are absorbed by active transport linked with Na^+ which moves down its concentration gradient. At the basal end of the cell transport into the cell is by passive or facilitated diffusion into the capillaries.

Vitamins

These are categorized into water soluble B and C; and fat soluble ADEK. Fat soluble vitamins follow fat absorption. Water soluble vitamins pass into the cells by mediated transport or passive diffusion.

B_{12} must bind to intrinsic factor (produced by parietal cells of stomach). When bound it attaches to epithelial cells in the ileum and is absorbed by endocytosis.

Minerals

Iron has to be in ferrous form Fe^{2+} to be absorbed. It forms soluble complexes, e.g. with ascorbate. It enters the villi cells by a protein carrier, is bound to ferritin once inside the cell and then a further carrier protein transports it across the cell membrane to the capillaries.

Calcium is absorbed by channels or carriers along the concentration gradient. Active transport (largely vitamin D dependent) also occurs in the duodenum and upper jejunum to take it across the cell membrane to the capillaries.

Problems with diet and nutrition

Overweight and obesity

Overall average weight has been increasing over several decades but now the UK has the highest level of obesity in Western Europe.

Obesity is closely linked with deprivation, especially among children, being more common in poor communities. While the aetiology may seem obvious (excess of energy intake over energy use) there are many risk factors including: genetics, sleep deprivation, bacterial gut flora, and viral infection. Blaming the individual for being overweight is unhelpful and inappropriate. At a societal level many factors contribute including: sedentary lifestyle, stress, and the availability and promotion of energy-dense foods. Excess weight increases the risk of coronary heart disease, hypertension, liver disease, osteoarthritis, stroke, type 2 diabetes, and some cancers (e.g. breast, colon, endometrial, and kidney). Body mass index (BMI) is a measure of weight status and is calculated by dividing a person's weight in kilograms by the square of their height in metres, i.e.:

$$\frac{body\ weight\,(kg)}{height^2\,(m^2)}$$

BMI 25–29.9 is overweight; BMI 30+ is obese.

Prevention for individuals is by limiting intake of energy-dense foods and being physically active but addressing the obesity trend will require society as a whole to think differently and for the environment and culture to promote healthier eating and physical activity.

Management includes: dietary interventions, physical activity, drugs to limit fat absorption, and bariatric surgery if severe.

Clinical relevance
- Many dental chairs have a weight limit of around 140 kg (23 stones)
- Staff may need training in manual handling
- Intravenous sedation and general anaesthesia (GA) will be more difficult, e.g. airway management, IV cannulation
- Medical history should be carefully checked for: hypertension, cardiovascular disease, diabetes mellitus, GORD (gastro-oesophageal reflux disease), osteoarthritis, gallstones, infection, and delayed wound healing.

Eating disorders

These are more common in women than in men. Triggers may include: genetic predisposition, hormonal factors, and psychological and cultural factors. There are 3 main types of clinical eating disorder.

Anorexia nervosa
Self-induced weight loss, distorted body image and fear of being fat (may cause amenorrhoea in females). Patients may also be prone to excessive exercise, vomiting/laxative/diuretic use. There is low body weight and low BMI.

Bulimia nervosa

Binge eating plus excessive exercise, vomiting/laxative/diuretic use.
Weight is in the normal range.

Binge eating disorder (compulsive eating)

This is probably the most common of the eating disorders.

Complications of recurrent vomiting include: electrolyte imbalance, alkalosis, potassium depletion, and risk of cardiac arrhythmia.

Suicide is a potential risk of anorexia.

Oral complications include: parotid gland swelling and dental erosion.

Management is by psychiatric support, dietetic support, and medical care to manage any complications.

Clinical relevance

Tooth surface loss (TSL) from repeated vomiting may be the first sign of an eating disorder. The clinician should be vigilant for the first signs of TSL and seek to find a cause. Most commonly patients will be reluctant to admit to self-induced vomiting. Obvious signs of being underweight may give a clue. Enquiry might be made sensitively about past and present slimming habits and whether eating is an issue. Liaison and referral with general medical practitioner is needed.

Practical advice to limit further damage includes:

• Fluoride mouthrinse prior to vomiting
• Delay brushing for at least an hour after vomiting
• After vomiting, use fluoride mouth rinse with low erosive potential
• Avoid acidic drinks.

Temporomandibular joint and surrounding musculature

The muscles of mastication 40
Lateral pterygoid muscle 44
The suprahyoid muscles 46
Structure and function of the temporomandibular joint 48
Treatment for temporomandibular disorders 50
The occlusion 52
Clinical considerations in occlusion 54
The jaw reflexes 56
Physiology of motor reflexes 58
How do muscles function? 60

The muscles of mastication

Mastication involves the coordinated movement of the mandible by its associated musculature that results in grinding and incising of food. The mandible moves at the temporomandibular joint.

The muscles are:
- The masseter muscles
- The temporalis muscle
- The medial and lateral pterygoid muscles
- The digastric muscles.

The motor innervation of the anterior belly of the digastric, masseter, temporalis, and pterygoid muscles is supplied by the mandibular division of the trigeminal nerve. The posterior belly of the digastric muscle is supplied by the facial nerve.

The masseter muscle

This muscle elevates the mandible (➲ See Fig. 2.1).
- Origin at the zygomatic arch
- Inserts into the angle and lateral surface of the mandible.

The temporalis muscle

Its main function is to elevate the mandible (➲ See Fig. 2.2).
- Origin from the temporal fossa
- Inserts into the mandibular coronoid process and anterior border of ramus.

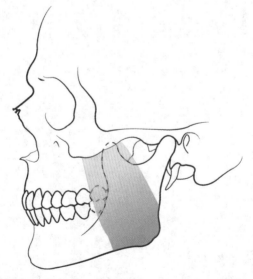

Fig. 2.1 The masseter muscle.

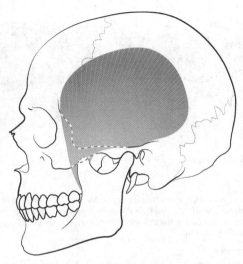

Fig. 2.2 The temporalis muscle attaches to the coronoid process of the mandible.

Medial pterygoid muscle

The main bulk of the medial pterygoid elevates the mandible, protrudes it and also moves it medially (➔ See Fig. 2.3)

• Origin at the medial surface of the lateral pterygoid plate
• Inserts into the medial surface of the angle of the mandible.

The small inferior head of the medial pterygoid muscle:

• Origin at the maxillary tuberosity and the pyramidal process of the palatine bone
• Fuses with the main bulk of the medial pterygoid to insert into the angle of the mandible.

Clinical significance of elevator muscle hyperactivity

Williamson and Lundquist[1] showed that when the posterior teeth are not in contact during lateral movements, the activity recorded by the elevator muscles is much reduced. Therefore, the effect of interfering posterior occlusal contacts will result in increased activity of the elevator muscles. This may have a damaging effect on the posterior teeth or the temporomandibular joint. The teeth, condyle, and muscular environment must work in harmony. Mongini showed that the occlusion and muscle function determine condylar remodelling, which results in changes in its shape[2]. The effect of experimentally introducing premature contacts during chewing is

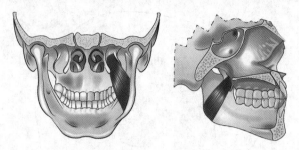

Fig. 2.3 Medial pterygoid muscle.

to cause a worsening of the masticatory performance[3]. Premature contacts must be avoided when providing new restorations for patients as they can result in the restoration fracturing, or the masseter or temporalis musculature becoming painful.

References

1   Williamson EH, Lundquist DO. (1983) Anterior guidance: its effect on electromyographic activity of the temporal and masseter muscles. *J Prosthet Dent* **49**:816–23.
2   Mongini F Anatomic and clinical evaluation of the relationship between the temporomandibular joint and occlusion. (1977) *J Prosthet Dent* **38**:539–51.
3   Eberhard L, Braun S, Wirth A, Schindler HJ, Hellmann D, Giannakopoulos NN. The effect of experimental balancing interferences on masticatory performance. *J Oral Rehabil* 2014; **41**:346–52.

Lateral pterygoid muscle

The lateral pterygoid muscle has two origins which join midway to form a central tendon that inserts into the base of the condyle.

The superior head acts to close the jaw and stabilize the condyle.
• Origin of the superior head of the lateral pterygoid muscle is the infratemporal surface of the greater wing of the sphenoid
• The superior head also inserts into the capsule and disc[4].

The inferior head acts to open the mouth by pulling the mandible forward.
• Origin of the inferior head is the lateral surface of the lateral pterygoid plate (➲ See Fig. 2.4)
• Insertion of the inferior head is the pterygoid fossa (the anteromedial surface of the condylar neck).

Clinical significance of lateral pterygoid function

• The two heads of the condyle act antagonistically with the superior head tending to close the jaw while the inferior head opens the jaw.

The inferior head of the lateral pterygoid muscle is active during jaw opening and the superior head during jaw closing and ipsilateral jaw movements. There is little evidence that variation in the insertion pattern of the superior head of the lateral pterygoid muscle is associated with internal derangement of the condylar disc.

The superior head of the lateral pterygoid is active during chewing, swallowing, and clenching of the teeth when it exerts a stabilizing action on the condyle.

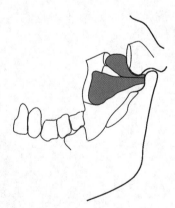

Fig. 2.4 Origin and insertion of the lateral pterygoid muscle.

Fracture of the condyle

Following fracture of the condylar neck, the anteromedial pull of the lateral pterygoid muscle displaces the condylar bone fragment. Necrosis of the condyle following fracture is rare because of the good blood supply.

The articular disc and condylar cartilage

Experiments in the porcine joint have shown that the collagen fibres of the surface fibrous zone of the condylar cartilage and the articular disc are arranged in an anteroposterior direction, making the tissue well adapted to resisting shear loads in this direction.

Articular disc

- Composed of thick posterior and anterior regions with a thinner middle region which is avascular
- Displacement of the disc causes locking and clicking of the joint.

Condylar cartilage

Major constituent is collagen.

The condylar cartilage in the temporo-mandibular joint has 4 distinct layers:

- The fibrous zone adjacent to the joint cavity
- Proliferative zone
- Mature zone
- Hypertrophic zone which lies on top of the subchondral bone of the condyle.

Osteoarthritis

- Associated with degeneration of the condylar cartilage
- Radiographic changes in the condyle are seen, e.g. flattening of the condylar surface and sclerosis of the bone. The mandibular ramus becomes shortened with changes in the occlusion.
- Repair of condylar cartilage is limited because the tissue has no blood vessels or nerves.

Reference

[4] Imanimoghaddam M, Madani AS, Hashemi EM. (2013) The evaluation of lateral pterygoid muscle pathologic changes and insertion patterns in temporomandibular joints with or without disc displacement using magnetic resonance imaging. *Int J Oral Maxillofac Surg*; **42**:1116–20.

The suprahyoid muscles

The digastric muscle

The digastric muscle is formed from an anterior and a posterior belly, with an intermediate tendon connecting both. The tendon is held in place by a fibrous sling which is attached to the hyoid bone. The function of the digastric muscle is to open the jaw with the infrahyoid muscles stabilizing the hyoid bone in position.

- Origin is the digastric notch on the medial surface of the mastoid process of the temporal bone
- Inserts into the digastric fossa close to the midline of the mandible.

In general, the muscles of mastication (masseter, temporalis, and pterygoid muscles) are supplied by the mandibular division of the trigeminal nerve with the exception of the digastric muscle. The anterior belly of the digastric is supplied by the trigeminal nerve but the posterior belly is supplied by the facial nerve.

Other suprahyoid muscles

Comprise the:
- Stylohyoid muscle
- Mylohyoid muscle
- Geniohyoid muscle.

See Fig. 2.5

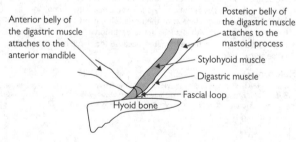

Anterior belly of the digastric muscle attaches to the anterior mandible

Posterior belly of the digastric muscle attaches to the mastoid process

Stylohyoid muscle

Digastric muscle

Fascial loop

Hyoid bone

Fig. 2.5 The stylohyoid muscle tendon embraces the digastric muscle.

Stylohyoid muscle
The stylohyoid muscle functions to retract the hyoid bone up and back and is active in swallowing.
• Origin is the styloid process
• Inserts into the greater cornu of the hyoid bone.

Mylohyoid muscle
The mylohyoid muscle elevates the tongue during swallowing of food.
• Origin is the mylohyoid ridge on both sides of the mandible.

The anterior fibres interdigitate to form a midline raphe.
• The posterior fibres insert into the hyoid bone.

Geniohyoid muscle
When the mandible is held in a fixed position by other muscles, the geniohyoid depresses the mandible and opens the jaw. The geniohyoid muscle is antagonistic to the stylohyoid muscle, because it pulls it forwards and upwards.
• Origin is the inferior genial tubercle on the symphysial surface of the mandible
• Inserts into the body of the hyoid bone.

The ligaments

These comprise the:
• Stylomandibular ligament: fascia that extends from the styloid process of the temporal bone to the angle of the mandible
• Stylohyoid ligament: fibrous band that extends from the styloid process to the lesser cornu of the hyoid bone.

Structure and function of the temporomandibular joint

The joint

- The articulatory surface of the temporomandibular joint is composed of fibrocartilage.
- The fibrocartilaginous articulatory disc divides the joint into an upper and lower compartment and is attached to the medial and lateral poles of the condylar process.
- Temporomandibular disorders are a result of the joint being unable to adapt to increased loading of the joint tissues, e.g. due to parafunction.
- The disc is avascular and without nervous innervation in the area in contact with the condyle.
- Posteriorly, the disc is thickened, highly vascular, and has a rich sensory innervation (bilaminar zone).
- Anteriorly, the superior head of the lateral pterygoid muscle inserts into the capsule and the disc.

The movements of the temporomandibular joint

When the jaw begins to open, the condyle rotates beneath the articular disc. The rotation occurs until the incisors are separated by about 12 mm. With further opening, the condyle and disc translate or move forward together onto the articular eminence.

Rotation of the condyle

The mandible can undergo a rotatory movement from 'centric relation', a position where the condyle abuts against the thinnest region of the articular disc. There are numerous, differing anatomical definitions of centric relation, but it is determined clinically by gently manipulating the mandible in a superior and anterior direction.

Translatory movement of the condyle

In the fully open position, the articular disc and condyle are positioned below the articular eminence with the tissues from the posterior-lateral region of the disc also pulled forwards. Further jaw opening is limited by the temporomandibular ligament which surrounds the temporo-mandibular joint. This ligament attaches to the outer surface of the articular eminence and runs obliquely downwards to connect with the lateral pole of the condyle.

The muscles responsible for elevating the mandible

These are the bilateral temporalis muscles, masseters, and medial pterygoid muscles.

The muscles that depress the mandible

These are the bilateral lateral pterygoid muscles and infra and suprahyoid muscles.

The muscles that protrude the mandible

These are the lateral pterygoid and medial pterygoid muscles acting together.

The muscles that move the mandible laterally

When moving the mandible to one side (e.g. the left side), the medial and lateral pterygoid muscles on the right side are active and vice versa. There would appear to be minor contributions from other muscles (e.g. masseter). Experimental evidence for the major contribution from the lateral pterygoid muscle was presented by Murray et al (1999)[5].

Clinical significance of lateral mandibular movements

The side to which the mandible moves in lateral jaw excursions is called the working side and the opposite side is called the non-working side. Bennett movement or mandibular side shift is a small lateral shift of the condyle on the working side during sideways movements of the mandible. It is the result of movement of the non-working side condyle to which it is joined. The orbiting non-working side condyle moves downwards and medially and its movement is limited by the shape of the mandibular condyle and fossa and the temporomandibular ligament.

Bilateral balanced occlusion

This occlusion is limited to complete dentures only. In lateral movements of the jaw, the denture teeth are arranged so that a maximum number remain in contact.

The natural dentition

In the natural dentition, the teeth in contact during lateral jaw movements ideally include only those teeth on the side to which the mandible moves. Group function occurs on the working side when there is a shared guidance with a number of teeth. No teeth on the nonworking side are in contact. In canine guidance, the canines on the working side disclude all of the other teeth during lateral jaw movements. This prevents lateral stress in the other teeth.

Reference

[5] Murray GM, Orfanos T, Chan JY, Wanigaratne K, Klineberg IJ. (1999) Electromyographic activity of the human lateral pterygoid muscle during contralateral and protrusive jaw movements. *Arch Oral Biol* **44**,: 269–85.

Treatment for temporomandibular disorders

Normal disc position

The disc of the temporomandibular joint is biconcave and is composed of a thick posterior band which normally sits on top of the mandibular condyle and a thinner intermediate zone located in a more anterior position. The disc has a shock-absorbing function. Anterior displacement of the disc can cause functional impairment to the joint.

Clinical signs and symptoms

Patients can present with:
• Pain
• Limitation in mouth opening (trismus)
• Clicking
• Occlusal changes.

Clinical diagnosis

Internal derangement of the temporomandibular joint occurs when the articular disc fails to function in harmony with the mandibular movements. Clicking may be associated with lateral deviation of the mandible during opening.

Disc displacement with reduction

The articular disk is displaced forward but on opening the disc returns to its normal position over the condylar head, accompanied by a 'popping' sound.

Treatment may involve jaw exercises or cognitive behavioural therapy. The latter is designed to help the patient to identify and re-evaluate stressful situations and assist in developing their coping skills. This is often followed by an upper acrylic stabilization splint therapy. This provides:
• Even bilateral occlusal contact after closure
• With lateral excursions of the mandible only the lower canines are in contact with the appliance.

Disc displacement without reduction (can be painful locking),

The articular disk has displaced forward so that it can no longer move back into place over the condyle during opening. No clicking sounds are heard. The forward movement of the condyle is prevented so jaw opening is restricted. This may be associated with pain in the area of the temporomandibular joint:
• If the condition occurs unilaterally, the mandible is deviated towards the affected side during opening movements
• Forward displacement of the condylar disc can be seen using magnetic resonance imaging.

It is recommended that patients receive education about their condition and that treatment is conservative. Most treatments (e.g. physiotherapy, splints, early mandibular manipulation, non-steroidal anti-inflammatory drugs [NSAIDs]) have some success in reducing symptoms.

Stabilization splint therapy

Patients with pain should be referred for treatment at an early stage to prevent the development of chronic symptoms. There is no evidence that occlusal adjustment of the teeth is effective in the treatment of temporo-mandibular disorders.

Splints are made to cover the occlusal surfaces of the teeth.

Temporomandibular disorders have a multifactorial aetiology and there-fore splints may work in a variety of different ways:

- They reduce the painful elevator musculature activity which has the effect of reducing electromyographic activity and myofascial pain. This will protect the temporomandibular joint from overloading.
- They provide an occlusion without any interference, allowing the muscles to function in harmony.
- Splint therapy also induces cortical thickening and positive bone remodelling in the condyle of those patients with osteoarthritis[6].

Anterior repositioning splint

This splint is used to treat an anteriorly displaced disc that is able to reduce (i.e. return to its normal position between the condylar head and articular eminence during opening). The effect of the splint is to cause a significant reduction in the muscle activity of the masseter and temporalis muscles and it may cause a repositioning of the displaced disc. The anteriorly positioned mandible also prevents articular disc trapping.

- There is some controversy as to whether the anterior positioning of the condyle with this splint is successful in allowing the non-reducing disc to assume its normal position above the condyle during opening. According to some authors, the non-reducing disc remains displaced anteriorly and the relief from symptoms is due to healing of the retro-discal tissues following the anterior condylar positioning.
- The clicking noise from the joint can be reduced or eliminated, but many symptoms can recur when the treatments stops and the appliance is not worn. The beneficial effects are often short-lived. With continuous, long-term wear, significant occlusal disorders develop (such as anterior open bite).

Reference

6   Ok SM, Lee J, Kim YI, Lee JY, Kim KB, Jeong SH. (2014) Anterior condylar remodeling observed in stabilization splint therapy for temporomandibular joint osteoarthritis. *Oral Surg Oral Med Oral Pathol Oral Radiol* **118**: 363–70.

The occlusion

The masticatory force should ideally be directed down the long axis of the teeth. Therefore when the patient protrudes their mandible with the teeth in contact, there are no interfering occlusal contacts with the posterior teeth. This avoids damaging lateral loads being applied to the posterior teeth in protrusive movements.

Mutually protected occlusion

The anterior teeth disclude the posterior teeth during dynamic movements and the posterior teeth provide protection of the anterior teeth by providing a stable occlusal vertical dimension. The disclusion of the posterior teeth during lateral and protrusive movements ensures that there are no damaging lateral loads on the periodontium of the posterior teeth, and the risk of posterior tooth wear and temporomandibular disorders is prevented.

The simultaneous contact of the teeth in maximum intercuspation (or intercuspal position) ensures that occlusal load is evenly spread throughout the dentition.

Non-working side contacts

Normally, the movement of the mandible is guided posteriorly by the condyle on the non-working side moving down the articular fossa. If two posterior teeth on the non-working side come into contact during this movement, then because they are close to the moving condyle, they can adversely guide or 'interfere' with its movement. This contact is termed a 'non-working side occlusal interference'. These interferences can guide the mandibular movement. In other words, the guidance can be transferred to the interfering tooth contact.

If these teeth are prepared for crowns, the interfering contacts are removed and the movement of the mandible is changed. However, the replacement crown may re-introduce the interfering contact and the patient may find it difficult to adapt to this.

Chewing

Rhythmic chewing can result from electrical activity generated in the brain stem, analogous to the rhythmic activity that results in breathing.

The activity is modified by sensory feedback from mechanoreceptors in the teeth and mucosa. Stimulation of the cortex in anaesthetized animals can cause a constant, alternating activity in the motor nerves of the mylohyoid and masseter muscles. Stimulating the sensory-motor cortex (in the absence of any phased sensory afferent input) can produce a rhythmic opening and closing jaw movement.
- The site of the rhythmic pattern generator in chewing is the medial bulbar reticular formation.
- The pattern generator is bilateral with the main control of the masticatory muscles originating from the contralateral cortex.
- The medial reticular formation controls the trigeminal motoneurons either directly or through pre-motoneurons situated close to the trigeminal nuclei or rostral lateral reticular formation.

The trigeminal nuclei

Sensory nerve fibres in the trigeminal nerve terminate in the main sensory nucleus, the spinal tract nucleus, or the mesencephalic nucleus. The nerves from the motor nucleus supply the muscles of mastication, tensor tympani, and tensor veli palatini. The buccinator muscle is supplied by the facial nerve.

The mesencephalic nucleus receives proprioceptive inputs from the temporo-mandibular joint, jaw muscle spindles, and periodontal ligament proprioceptors.

- Neurons of the mesencephalic nucleus project to the trigeminal motor nucleus where they form synaptic connections with the masticatory muscle motoneurons.
- Neurons from the pre-frontal cortex have been found in rats to project onto the mesencepahalic nucleus, and by adjusting the sensory input therefore may modify the elevator jaw muscle activity.
- Nerve fibres from the mesencephalic nucleus project sensory fibres to the posterior hypothalamus. Bilateral lesions of the mesencephalic nucleus in mice result in changes in feeding behaviour.

The spinal tract nucleus receives pain and temperature sensation from sensory afferent fibres which cross the midline and ascend to the thalamus in the ventral trigeminal tract, with further relays to the somato-sensory area of the cortex. Damage to the sensory root will result in loss of ipsilateral pain and temperature sensation.

The main sensory nucleus receives tactile sensory input. The majority of fibres cross the midline to ascend to the thalamus, but some remain ipsilateral and ascend in the dorsal trigeminal tract. Tumours involving the main sensory nucleus will produce decreased tactile sensation in the face.

The motor nuclei supplies the following muscles:

- The masseter muscle
- Temporalis muscle
- Medial and lateral pterygoid muscles
- Mylohyoid muscle
- And the anterior belly of the digastric.

When there has been unilateral sectioning of the mandibular motor root, the mandible deviates towards the paralysed side during opening, due to the activity of the medial and lateral pterygoid muscles.

Clinical considerations in occlusion

Rest position

This is the position adopted by the mandible when the patient is at rest and is determined by the mandibular muscle activity and its visco-elastic properties. Both elevator and depressor muscles are minimally active. It is of importance to determine this position when constructing complete dentures so that adequate space can be created between the denture teeth when the patient is at rest. The patient should have their head in an upright position when assessing rest position.

Interocclusal rest space (freeway space)

This is the distance between the teeth when the patient's mandible is in the rest position. This is determined by placing small pencil marks on the nose and chin and separately measuring:

• The distance between the marks with the patient biting their teeth together (occlusal vertical dimension) and
• The distance between the marks when the patient's mandible is in the rest position (rest vertical dimension).

The interocclusal rest space is calculated as the difference between these two measurements.

Measuring the interocclusal rest space in the edentulous patient

In this situation, an amount of interocclusal rest space (usually 2–4 mm) is incorporated in the new complete dentures. Using markers on the nose and chin, the correct occlusal vertical dimension can be determined.

Maximal intercuspal position (MIP)

The teeth are in complete intercuspation.

Condylar guidance

This is the regulation of the mandibular movements by the condyle.

Anterior (or incisal) guidance

Anterior guidance is the regulation of the mandibular movement described by the contacting anterior teeth. The anterior guidance allows the posterior teeth to separate during lateral movements of the jaw. If a patient moves their mandible to their left side, the right side of their mandible is the non-working side and the left side is the working side. Similarly, if they move their mandible to their right, the right side becomes the working side and the left the non-working side. New restorations should function in harmony with the existing anterior guidance (conformative approach) or where the existing maximal intercuspal position is unsatisfactory then the occlusion should be re-organized.

In chewing movements, there is an inferior movement of the mandible followed by a lateral movement to the side on which the food is located. The teeth penetrate the food. The mandible returns to the maximal inter-cuspal position.

In Fig. 2.6 position M represents the retruded contact position, i.e. the occlusal relationship that occurs at the most retruded position of the

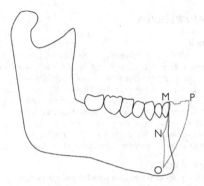

Fig. 2.6 The extreme border movements of the mandible (M, N, O, P) as traced out by the lower incisor teeth in the sagittal plane.

condyles in the joint cavities. During separation of the teeth (moving from position M to N), the lower incisors move in a movement arc with the centre of rotation at the condyle. Further opening causes the condyle to translate forwards with the lower incisors moving to a position O in maximal opening. The axis of rotation is in the ramus of the mandible. Position P is the position of the lower incisors at maximal protrusion with the teeth in contact.

Articulators

These devices are used in the clinic and laboratory to simulate the movements of the mandible to a varying extent, depending on their complexity.

- The hinge articulator relates the maxillary and mandibular casts in their maximal intercuspal position
- The average value articulator has a fixed condylar guidance, usually about 25°.
- A semi-adjustable articulator used with a facebow recording allows the reproduction of the terminal hinge movement of the mandible during closure
- Fully adjustable articulator.

The jaw reflexes

The jaw jerk
When a downward tap is delivered to the chin with the jaw held slightly open, there is a reflex contraction of the masseter followed by mandibular closure. This fast, monosynaptic reflex is not much affected by blocking the mechanoreceptor input from the teeth (i.e. by using local anaesthetic). The tap to the jaw stimulates the muscle spindles in the elevator muscles causing afferent stimulation, which enters the motor root (not the sensory root) of the trigeminal nerve passing to the mesencepahalic nucleus. Axons from the mesencepahlic nucleus enter the trigeminal motor nucleus where there is a monosynaptic relay, followed by stimulation of the jaw elevator muscles.

Unloading reflex
When biting tough food, the muscle spindles provide excitatory input to the motoneurons so that the muscle force increases. When the food eventually breaks, the muscle shortens and the stimulatory activity from the muscle spindles ceases. The closing muscle activity is quickly reduced. This occurs because the tension in the muscle spindles is reduced by the extrafusal muscle continuing to shorten. There is a reduction in the Ia afferent activity to the trigeminal mesencephalic nucleus and the muscle activity closing the jaw.

Tonic activity in the jaw opening muscles is also important in preventing sudden collision of the teeth. Should the teeth occlude suddenly then the periodontal receptors will act to inhibit motoneuron activation of the jaw elevator muscles.

Clinical significance
- The jaw jerk reflex is exaggerated in central lesions above the pons, e.g. pseudobulbar palsy affecting the corticobulbar tract (motoneurones connecting the cerebral cortex with the brainstem).
- Trigeminal neuralgia is a sudden intense pain that lasts a few seconds and can be initiated by gently touching the trigger zone. The cause of trigeminal neuralgia is thought to be related to the pressure of the intracranial blood vessels on the nerve. Other diseases can give similar pain symptoms of trigeminal neuralgia and include multiple sclerosis or tumours. Patients should therefore undergo a neurological assessment. Carbamazepine (an anti-convulsant) is the main treatment for trigeminal neuralgia.
- When the mandible is held in its resting position, there is typically a space between the occlusal surfaces of the upper and lower teeth of about 3–8 mm. This space must be maintained when complete dentures are constructed to allow good function and aesthetics. When the dentist records the rest position in the clinic, it is the visco-elastic properties of the peri-oral tissues which maintain the rest position and not the stretch reflex.

Human jaw muscle physiology
When a tap is delivered to the chin with the subject clenching their teeth, the reflex excitation to the elevator muscles is overlaid by a depression of the elevator muscle activity (called a 'silent period').

Clinical significance

- The duration of the silent period is increased in those with temporo-mandibular disorders (also called temporo-mandibular dysfunction). This cannot be used as a clinical diagnostic tool as the reported silent period is very variable and is strongly affected by anticipation of the chin tap.
- The importance of the jaw jerk is that it measures the function of the sensory and motor aspects of the trigeminal nerve and is unaffected by any functional loss in the higher centres.
- Multiple sclerosis is a demyelination of nerves that affects the CNS. A delayed or abnormal jaw reflex test is not always found in patients suspected of multiple sclerosis with brainstem involvement.

There is no jaw opening reflex when an upward tap is delivered to the mandible. There is little anatomical evidence for the presence of muscle spindles in the human anterior digastric muscle.

The function of periodontal receptors

The function of periodontal receptors is critical to the chewing of food between the teeth. These receptors signal the mechanical properties of the food. They do this because there are two main populations of receptors; those responding to change at low levels of forces only and a minority that respond in a linear manner to increasing loads up to high levels of force. Input from the periodontal receptors will allow the selection of the most appropriate force levels to be applied to the food as it softens and comminutes during chewing.

The jaw-opening muscles do not have muscle spindles. This function is provided by periodontal mechanoreceptors providing information about the resistance

Physiology of motor reflexes

Muscle spindle reflexes

Because intrafusal fibres run in parallel with the rest of the muscle, they are stretched by tapping a muscle tendon. When stretched, the intrafusal fibres stimulate the group IA afferent neurons in the central non-contractile region. They stimulate the α-motoneurons to contract the muscle in a monosynaptic reflex.

- The contractile parts at either end of the intrafusal fibres are innervated by γ motoneurons. These neurons match the length of the intrafusal and extrafusal muscle fibres. They make the intrafusal muscle fibres able to respond despite changes in length of the extrafusal muscle fibres.
- Type II afferent fibres also innervate the muscle spindle. They respond to static muscle length.
- Muscle spindles are arranged in parallel to the rest of the muscle.

Golgi tendon organ reflexes

Golgi tendon organs are arranged in series with the rest of the muscle. When muscle tension rises, the Golgi tendon organs are activated.

- They are innervated by afferent type IB sensory nerve fibres which synapse with interneurons.
- Muscle tension is reduced by interneuron inhibition of the α-motoneuron.

Each tendon organ monitors muscle tension over several motor units.

What is the difference between Golgi tendon organ and the muscle spindle reflexes?

- With the Golgi tendon organ reflex, the reflex is polysynaptic (unlike the stretch reflex).
- Golgi tendon organs have no motor innervation.

Maintaining posture

When a commuter is pushed gently during a train journey, his or her muscle spindles are activated by the slight stretching movements. These activate the muscles of the legs to maintain an upright posture.

The intrafusal fibres

There are two main types of intrafusal fibres: the nuclear bag fibres and the nuclear chain fibres. The γ motoneurons excite the muscle spindles and keep them tense. In the absence of γ motoneuron activity, the spindles would be unable to detect the stretch of the extrafusal fibres and any fine movement would be lost.

Nuclear bag fibres

The nuclear bag fibres can be further sub-divided into static (b_2) and dynamic (b_1) bag fibres. The division has an anatomical basis as static bag fibres have an afferent innervation from groups IA and II myelinated nerve fibres, but dynamic bag fibres only have IA afferent innervation.

- The static (b_2) bag fibres respond to muscle length
- The dynamic (b_1) bag fibres respond to change in muscle length.

Nuclear chain fibres

These fibres receive efferent innervation via static γ-motoneurons and afferent innervation via groups II and IA neurons. They are thought to be mainly responsive to the length of the spindle.

In summary

Afferent innervation of spindles

Dynamic afferent innervation (group IA) mediates the monosynaptic stretch reflex. The static afferent fibres (group II) sense a step change in the length of the muscle and synapse with interneurons in the spinal cord.

Efferent innervation of spindles

The main role of the fusimotor efferent system is to allow the spindles to continue to provide sensory feedback to the motor cortex, particularly during a muscle contraction. Fusimotor activation during shortening of a muscle prevents the silencing of the afferent discharges.

Clinical significance

- Following a cerebro-vascular accident, the inhibitory function of the central nervous system on the stretch reflex may be reduced.
- Damage to the anterior horn cells will reduce or eliminate the muscle spindle reflex.
- Muscle tone is maintained by central stimulation of the γ motoneurons which in turn activates the nuclear chain fibres. These activate the spinal interneurons and alpha motoneurons controlling the extrafusal fibres, resulting in muscle contraction.

Central pattern generator (CPG)

Some evidence exists for a central pattern generator in the brainstem that is responsible for the rhythmic chewing movements in mastication.

- Stimulating the reticular formation of the midbrain can elicit chewing movements. The chewing CPG continues to function even on removal of the influences of higher centres or sensory feedback from the masticatory muscles.
- The chewing CPG may produce a rhythmic efferent activity, but the force applied to food must be influenced by the masticatory muscle reflexes, and the input from periodontal mechanoreceptors.

How do muscles function?

The neuromuscular junction

The action potential travelling down the motor nerve activates a set of muscle fibres (the motor unit). The number of muscle fibres in each motor unit varies between muscles and determines the force generated by that unit. The muscle fibres of the motor unit act in unison when activated by the motor nerve action potential.

Not all muscle fibres are the same; they differ according to speed of contraction and other properties (➡ See Table 2.1). Fibres are classified into type I and II according to their histochemical reaction.

The different properties of the muscle fibres is reflected in the differing muscle fibre structure; in general, type I fibres are rich in oxidative enzymes and react faintly to myofibrillar adenosine triphosphatase. Most human limb muscles contain mixtures of type I and type II fibres. The histochemical classification of a muscle fibre has some correspondence with the myosin isoform content (➡ See Table 2.1).

Jaw elevator muscles are mainly composed of type I fibres (and some type IIB fibres), with very few type IIA fibres present, but individual fibres can contain more than one type of myosin heavy chain isoform. This provides the muscle with considerable functional versatility.

Nerve and muscle function are closely intertwined

- The electromyographic activity in a muscle reflects its histochemical profile. Training can induce changes in composition of myosin heavy chain isoforms from a fast to slow type.[7]
- The process of atrophy that occurs in ageing muscle may be mainly caused by denervation and degeneration of neuromuscular junctions. There is a shift in elderly muscle towards the co-expression of fibres with myosin heavy chains I and IIA. There are fewer type IIX fibres.[8]

Table 2.1 Summary of muscle fibre characteristics

Property	Type I	Type IIA	Type IIB
Twitch speed	Slow	Fast	Fast
Fatigue	Resistant to fatigue	Resistant to fatigue	Fatigues quickly
Motor unit size	Small	Large	Large
Myosin heavy chain isoform	Type I	Type IIA	Types IIB and IIX
Fibre diameter	Small	Small	Largest

With low force effort, low threshold type I muscle fibres are recruited, but with the requirement for increasing intensity of effort, there is recruitment of Type IIA and finally Type IIB fibres. Type IIB fibres undergo preferential atrophy in disuse and also in the short-term atrophic changes observed in denervation. Human experiments that have tried to change the muscle fibre type through changes in activity have not been successful. However, animal experiments that have exchanged the innervation of muscles have produced changes in muscle composition; e.g. cross-reinnervated slow muscle gains the increased myosin ATPase activity of fast-muscle myosin.

A number of fibres in the jaw muscles contain a mixture of types of myosin chains; therefore the motoneuron activity may not be the only determinant of the type of myosin chain isoform. Muscle has been previously thought to be stable in structure with very little muscle fibre replacement, but the muscle fibres in the jaw may undergo continuous compositional change, perhaps through continual repair and maintenance.

Myogenic helix-loop-helix transcription factors (such as MyoD and Myogenin) have been put forward as regulators of muscle myosin heavy chain composition. They are thought to summate the electrical activity of the muscle and control the myosin gene expression. Cross innervation and denervation result in changes in both MyoP and Myogenin mRNA levels.

Jaw muscle activity and composition

In monkeys rendered edentulous, there was atrophy of type I fibres in the masseter and temporalis muscles, with an increased proportion of Type IIB fibres in the posterior masseter. Similar changes may occur in the elevator muscles of edentulous human patients, but any experimental studies would need sufficient number of subjects to account for the genetic variation between subjects.

- The composition of the masseter muscle varies between species and the reason for this is probably the differing predominant jaw muscle activity.

Reinnervation

After denervation, surgical nerve repair is successful with a recovery of function but after about a year, nerve repair has a much less certain prognosis. This is due to proliferation of the muscle connective tissue preventing the regenerating axons from making contact with the atrophied muscle fibres.

Muscle structure

The muscle fibre is composed of bundles of myofibrils, which have alternating dark (A band) and light (I bands). In the centre of the A-band is a dark Z disk. The functional unit of the myofibril is the sarcomere which is measured between successive Z-discs.

The myosin filaments are located entirely in the A-band. Thin actin filaments slide between the myosin filaments, increase the overlap of the two and generate the muscle tension. The H-band is that area of the A-band where the myosin is not overlapped by actin.

The neuromuscular junction

There is no electrical continuity between the nerve and the muscle membranes. The arrival of the action potential at the neuromuscular junction causes Ca^{2+} ions to diffuse into the axon from the extracellular fluid. This causes vesicles containing acetylcholine to fuse with the nerve membrane and discharge their contents into the gap between the nerve and the muscle membranes. The acetylcholine diffuses across the cleft, combines with receptors on the muscle membrane and causes an increased permeability to sodium and potassium ions. If the threshold is exceeded, an action potential is then generated along the muscle membrane.

Muscle function

Transverse tubules conduct the action potential from the muscle surface into the myofibril. Depolarization of the transverse tubules causes Ca^{2+} ion release from the terminal cisternae. The calcium (Ca^{2+}) ions bind to 'beads' of troponin on the thin filaments and expose the active site of actin which is then able to interact with the myosin. The binding site is activated by the activated troponin moving the inhibitory protein tropomyosin sideways so that myosin-actin cross bridges form. The binding of the globular myosin heads to the actin filament activates sliding and the release of adenosine diphosphate (ADP) and phosphate. Finally, the binding of adenosine triphosphate (ATP) to myosin causes the globular head to release the actin with movement of the globular myosin head. The movement during the attaching and detaching of a single myosin head is about 8–13 nm with about 8–12 pN generated.

Contraction stops when the Ca^{2+} ions are actively pumped back into the sarcoplasmic reticulum and tropomyosin returns to its inhibitory state, blocking the actin-binding site.

Diseases of muscle

Duchenne muscular dystrophy

It is a recessive, sex-linked genetic disorder affecting only males. The disease is caused by a mutation in dystrophin, a muscle protein. The absence of functional dystrophin causes membrane destabilization and changes in intracellular calcium movements. It causes muscle weakness and death usually occurs in the 20s due to myocardial fibrosis and cardiac hypertrophy.

Myotonic dystrophy

This is an autosomal-dominant disorder. There are two major classifications of myotonic dystrophy; type 1 (due to a mutation in the *DMPK* gene) and type 2 (due to mutations in the *CNBP* gene).

Clinical features include
• Ptosis
• Cataracts
• Muscle wasting.

Poliomyelitis

Clinical features are varied and may vary from mild cases of gastroenteritis to severe muscle atrophy (paralytic poliomyelitis). Paralytic poliomyelitis can involve the spine (spinal poliomyelitis), the brain stem (bulbar poliomyelitis), or both (bulbospinal poliomyelitis)

The virus enters the body through the oropharynx and multiplies in the local lymphoid tissues. Paralysis of limbs is caused by the virus entering the afferent nerves and causing destruction of the anterior horn cells in the spinal cord and/or brain cells.

Clinical features include:
- Fever at initial onset
- Can cause a flaccid muscular paralysis.

Regeneration of muscle following injury

A population of stem cells in the muscle, satellite cells, is responsible for regeneration of muscle following injury and cannot be replaced by other sources. Clinical trials of the satellite cells have been disappointing as a variety of different cells are probably necessary for promoting differentiation. As yet there is no cure for dystrophic muscle disease using stem cell technology.

Hypertrophy of muscle

Hypertrophy of muscle, as a result of exercise, results from the differentiation and proliferation of satellite cells. These cells then fuse with existing myofibres to produce additional muscle protein.

References

[7] Harridge SD, Andersen JL, Hartkopp A, Zhou S, Biering-Sørensen F, Sandri C, Kjaer M. (2002) Training by low-frequency stimulation of tibialis anterior in spinal cord-injured men. *Muscle Nerve* 25: 685–94.

[8] Rowan SL1, Rygiel K, Purves-Smith FM, Solbak NM, Turnbull DM, Hepple RT. Denervation causes fiber atrophy and myosin heavy chain co-expression in senescent skeletal muscle. (2012) *PLoS One.* 7:e29082.

Oral mucosa, saliva, and speech

Oral mucosa – normal structure and function 66
Oral ulceration 68
Cancer 70
Saliva 74
Swallowing 78
Speech 82

Oral mucosa – normal structure and function

Oral mucosa is categorized into three types:
- Lining mucosa which is freely mobile, loose, and non-keratinized
- Masticatory mucosa is tightly bound down to underlying bone and is keratinized. It covers hard palate, tongue dorsum, and gingiva. Cell turnover is slower than in lining mucosa. (➔ See Fig. 3.1 and Table 3.1)
- Specialized mucosa covers the tongue and has taste buds and lingual papillae.

Non-keratinized mucosa may transform to produce keratin in response to friction or chemical trauma and may produce excess keratin (hyperkeratinization). In some places there is no submucosa and the mucosa is tightly bound down to the periosteum. This is known as muco-periosteum, e.g. across much of the palate and the gingiva.

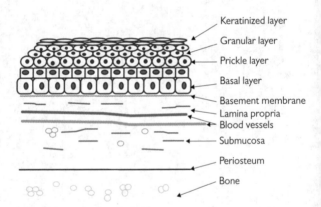

Keratinized layer
Granular layer
Prickle layer
Basal layer
Basement membrane
Lamina propria
Blood vessels
Submucosa
Periosteum
Bone

Fig. 3.1 Layers of keratinized oral mucosa.

Table 3.1 Structure for keratinized oral epithelium

Layer	Contents
Stratum corneum	Keratinized superficial layer of flattened non-vital squames on the epithelial surface
Stratum granulosum	Granular layer of keratinocytes in the stratum granulosum differentiating into nonvital surface cells
Stratum spinosum	Prickle layer of cells terminally differentiate as they migrate to the surface from the stratum basale
Stratum basale	Basal layer of cuboidal cells with most active cell division
Basement membrane	Lamina lucida, which is less dense and is toward the epithelial side Lamina densa, middle of the three parts Lamina reticularis, which is less dense than the lamina densa and is located next to the lamina propria Mechanical adhesions with the basal lamina is by hemidesmosomes
Lamina propria	Superficial layer of loose connective tissue Capillary plexus Dense deeper layer of fibres Fibrous connective tissue layer that consists of a network of collagen (types I and III) and elastin fibres in some regions The main cells of the lamina propria are the fibroblasts, which are responsible for the production of the fibres as well as the extracellular matrix.
Submucosa	May or may not be present Containing: loose connective tissue, adipose, connective tissue, salivary glands Fordyce spots are scattered throughout the non-keratinized tissue. They are deposits of sebum from misplaced sebaceous glands in the submucosa.

Oral ulceration

Ulceration is a break in the epithelium exposing the underlying connective tissue and possibly even deeper layers. There may be a red halo of inflammation around it and a yellow/grey necrotic centre. There are many potential causes.

1. Local causes: mechanical trauma and burns
2. Recurrent aphthous stomatitis (RAS)

RAS is a group of conditions where the immunological system becomes partly dysfunctional. The mildest forms are very common (affecting around 20%) and in many there is a genetic predisposition too. It is thought that there may be a cross-reaction between antigens in oral mucosa and microorganisms. T helper cells and some natural killer (NK) cells take part first, later followed by cytotoxic cells in an antibody dependent cellular cytotoxicity (ADCC) reaction.

3. Infections:
   • Viruses: herpes simplex, HIV, coxsackie, echovirus
   • Bacteria: acute necrotizing gingivitis, syphilis, tuberculosis
   • Fungi: deep mycoses—rare systemic fungal infection, often in immunocompromised patients
4. Drugs: cytotoxic drugs, nicorandil, NSAIDs, and many more
5. Systemic diseases
   • GI disorders: ulcerative colitis, coeliac, or Crohn's disease
   • Blood disorders: anaemia, haematinic deficiencies, leukaemia, neutropenia, lymphoid tissue disorders
   • Mucocutaneous disorders: lichen planus, pemphigus, pemphigoid
6. Malignant disease: an ulcer that lasts 2–3 weeks without healing after removal of any obvious local cause should be urgently investigated to exclude carcinoma
7. Autoimmune disorders, e.g. systemic lupus erythematosus (SLE), Behçet's syndrome, granulomatosis with polyangiitis
8. Idiopathic, e.g. necrotizing sialometaplasia

Behçet's syndrome

This syndrome is rare in the UK, but more common in the Mediterranean, Turkey, the Middle East, Japan, and south-east Asia. Genetic markers HLA-B51/HLA-B5 carry an increased risk and there is a familial clustering rather than direct inheritance. Symptoms start in the 20s–30s and include the following.

• Mouth ulcers frequent painful ulcers of the tongue and throat often of herpetiform type
• Genital ulcers
• Skin problems: boils, spots, red patches, ulcers
• Eye inflammation is of the uveal tract from iris to the retina and may result in loss of vision
• Extreme fatigue
• Joint pain and swelling
• Bowel symptoms: bloating, abdominal pain, diarrhoea
• Thrombosis in surface veins.

The aetiology is probably autoimmune with exposure to an infectious agent triggering a cross-reactive immune response. Some human heat shock proteins (HSPs) have been found to have 50% homology with mycobacterial HSP and a T-cell response has been elicited with exposure to both bacterial and human homogenates in Behçet syndrome patients. HSPs have been found in high concentrations in oral ulcers and active skin lesions in patients with Behçet. The pathology is two types of vascular damage—widespread vasculitic lesions with inflammatory infiltration by T cells and neutrophils, and thrombosis due to impaired fibrinolysis and pathologic activation of the procoagulant cascade via endothelial injury.

Kawasaki disease (KD)

This is a rare form of vasculitis which affects children under the age of 5 years with a higher risk in Asian children, e.g. Japanese and Koreans. Aetiology is uncertain but it seems to be an example of a destructive host response to a pathogen in a genetically susceptible host. Infection is thought to trigger the disease. The inhaled agent (probably viral) infects bronchial epithelial cells. An innate immune response is initiated and the agents engulfed by tissue macrophages are carried to local lymph nodes where they initiate the adaptive immune response. So macrophages, Ag-specific T cells, and IgA plasma cells infiltrate the bronchial epithelial cells. Circulating monocytes and macrophages containing the KD agent reach specific susceptible tissues (vascular and ductal tissues). Inflammatory mediators have been identified: vascular endothelial growth factor, matrix metalloproteinase, tumour necrosis factor-a (TNF-a), and other inflammatory cytokines. Muscle layers in arteries can be destroyed resulting in thinning and ballooning of the vessel walls leading to aneurysm. In the bronchial epithelium, the KD agent persists within cytoplasmic inclusion bodies that are shielded from the immune system.

Clinical features

Include: fever; rash; conjunctivitis; red, swollen, cracked lips; strawberry tongue; general erythema of oral mucosa; swollen hands and feet with redness of the palms; cervical lymphadenopathy; myocarditis, pericarditis, coronary artery aneurysms and stenosis.

Necrotizing sialometaplasia (NS)

This is a benign, self-limiting disorder of salivary glands mostly affecting the hard palate although it may occur wherever there are minor salivary glands. The lesion presents as a discrete swelling or ulcer which may or may not be painful. It mimics carcinoma both clinically and histologically.

Cancer

Also ➲ see Chapter 4 for bone cancer

How does cancer develop?

Oral cancer is caused by genetic aberrations resulting from an accumulation of damage to DNA due to exposure to environmental carcinogens. Several DNA mutations seem necessary before the cells and tissues affected change in their morphology and behaviour to a recognizably pre-malignant or potentially malignant cell. Genetic aberrations acquired during development of a cancer include loss or gain of genetic sequences on chromosomes or acquisition of DNA mutations. These specific DNA mutations lead to altered amino acids and thus change in cell proteins.

The progression from a normal cell to a potentially malignant cell and finally to a cancer cell is marked by an increase in cells escaping the normal growth control mechanisms, and then proliferating autonomously. The cells divide more and survive longer than normal, they lose cohesion and invade across the basement membranes and into the underlying tissues. This process may be referred to as oncogenesis or carcinogenesis.

A series of steps lead to the aberrant expression and function of molecules regulating cell signalling, growth, survival, motility, angiogenesis (blood vessel proliferation), and cell cycle control. Cell cycle control is disturbed particularly by oncogene over-expression or over-activity (amplification) which drives cell proliferation. So oncogenes, such as the epidermal growth factor receptor (EGFR) gene, may be potential targets for cancer therapy. Other genes are protective. For example, tumour suppressor genes (TSGs) have an anti-proliferative action. The proteins for which they code may have the effect of repressing the continuation of the cell cycle or promoting apoptosis of the damaged cell, and sometimes do both. Apoptosis is the organized destruction of a cell which is initiated by either a signal from a neighbouring cell or the cell itself due to sensed internal damage. This process does not cause an inflammatory response and is commonly referred to as programmed cell death.

The steps towards cancer are thus:
1. Mutagenic agent (free radicals: OH, NO) acts on DNA in basal cells
2. DNA mutation occurs and escapes DNA repair or TSG-initiated apoptosis
4. DNA mutation is not lethal for the cell
5. Mutated viable cell escapes the immune system

Potentially malignant lesions

Oral cancer may arise on previously normal mucosa but in some cases (perhaps around 50%) there are visible signs of changes that can signify an increased risk of cancer.

Leukoplakia

This is a predominantly white lesion of the oral mucosa that cannot be characterized as any other definable lesion. The appearance clinically is variable, histology shows a variable degree of dysplasia and there is a similar range of outcomes. Some may be early carcinoma when they first present but most never progress to carcinoma.

Table 3.2 Features of oral epithelial dysplasia

Intra-cellular changes	Epithelial architecture changes
• Cell and nuclear pleomorphism (variable size, shape and staining of cells and nuclei)	• Thickened epithelium
	• Hyperkeratosis
	• Basal cell hyperplasia
• Nuclear hyperchromatism (excessive nuclear staining)	• Loss of polarity
• Anisocytosis (cells of unequal sizes)	• Disordered maturation from basal to squamous cells
• Anisonucleosis (variation in the size of the cell nuclei)	• Bulbous drop-shaped rete pegs
	• Increased cellular density
• Increased and abnormal mitotic figures	• Dyskeratosis (premature keratinization and keratin pearls deep in epithelium)
• Enlarged nuclei and cells	• Acantholysis (loss of intercellular connections and resulting in loss of cohesion between cells)
Severe dysplasia	**Severe dysplasia**
• ↑ number and size of nucleoli	• Loss of stratification
• Apoptotic bodies	• Full thickness change

Erythroplakia

This is a predominantly red lesion of the oral mucosa that cannot be characterized as any other definable lesion. The risk of malignant transformation is around 90% and immediate excision is recommended.

Progression of lesions is difficult to predict and although much research is ongoing to find reliable markers for malignant transformation the histology is still the best predictor. A biopsy is checked for features of oral epithelial dysplasia and an assessment made of the degree of dysplasia—mild, moderate, or severe. (➲ See Table 3.2.)

How is oral mucosa affected by iron deficiency, alcohol, and smoking?

In patients with iron deficiency anaemia, there is a reduction in the total epithelial thickness of the buccal epithelium. This reduction in epithelial thickness occurs principally at the expense of the maturing cell layers. Alcohol appears to make the oral mucosa more permeable to the penetration of carcinogens and acts synergistically with tobacco and smokeless tobacco. The most important environmental risk factors for upper digestive tract cancers are tobacco smoking, alcohol intake, and poor oral hygiene. They all result in increased acetaldehyde (ACH) levels in saliva. Alcohol itself is not mutagenic but it is metabolized to mutagenic ACH. In addition, some alcoholic drinks contain high ACH concentrations as a congener. Many oral microbes possess alcohol dehydrogenase enzyme activity (e.g. *Neisseria, Streptococci, Candida*) and have been shown to be able to produce carcinogenic amounts of ACH from ethanol or glucose. Smoking is also a major

risk factor for chronic periodontal disease and also worsens treatment outcomes and wound healing. Vasoconstriction and impaired polymorphonuclear leucocyte (PMN) function are thought to be the main reasons.

Diagnosis and management of oral cancers

Every dental examination should include extra-oral soft tissues, including
regional lymph nodes and intraoral soft tissue. Any suspect lesions should
be assessed and suspected cancer pathway referral (i.e. with the patient
seen by a secondary care clinician within 2 weeks) should follow if any of
the following features are present:

• Unexplained ulceration in the oral cavity lasting for more than 3 weeks
• A persistent and unexplained lump in the neck
• A lump on the lip or in the oral cavity consistent with oral cancer
• A red or red and white patch in the oral cavity consistent with
  erythroplakia or erythroleukoplakia.

See NICE guideline [NG12] (2015)[1].

Diagnosis is mostly by biopsy. If the lesion is small, an excisional biopsy is
preferred, i.e. complete removal of the lesion, with a border of normal tissue. Otherwise incisional biopsy is used to remove a representative sample
from the lesion. The sample is examined for signs of histopathology, as in
Table 3.2. If the diagnosis is confirmed further investigation will be needed
to plan the management.

Management of oral cancer requires a multi-professional team and is
primarily by surgery with or without radiotherapy to control the primary
tumour and any lymph nodes metastases.

How does oral cancer spread?

Spread of the cancer happens:

• By lymphatics to regional lymph nodes
• By the bloodstream to lung, brain, liver and elsewhere
• By local spread, may damage and cause dysfunction in vital organs,
  resulting in pain and other symptoms (dysarthria, dysphagia, tooth
  mobility).

Radiation-induced oral mucositis

This is a common complication of radiotherapy in the head and neck
because of the high turnover of oral mucosal cells (7–14 day cycle). Painful
erythematous and ulcerative lesions can be severe, affect the patient's ability to eat and their nutritional status. Mucositis can thus be a dosage-limiting
factor in radiotherapy. Mucositis is especially likely to occur if the target
tumour is in the oral cavity or pharynx and if concomitant chemotherapy is
given. Mucositis may be complicated by local infections, especially in immu-
nosuppressed patients.

Mechanism of action

This is by direct damage to basal epithelial cells. DNA damage can result in cell
death or injury. Non-DNA injury is initiated through a variety of mechanisms,
some of which are mediated by the generation of reactive oxygen species
(damaging, unstable, reactive molecules containing oxygen). Macrophages produce inflammatory cytokines (e.g. TNF-α and interleukin-6). These mediators

also have a positive-feedback loop that amplifies the original effect. The commensal flora of the oropharynx may also be directly affected by the radiation, reducing the flora's resistance to colonization by pathogens.

Management of oral mucositis

This is by:

- Nutritional support with a soft or liquid diet (gastrostomy tube if severe)
- Good oral hygiene using soft toothbrush, flossing, and bland rinses (saline or sodium bicarbonate rinses): note that chlorhexidine is no longer recommended
- Management of dry mouth with sips of water, artificial saliva products, sugarless gum, or cholinergic agents
- Therapeutic interventions – low-level laser treatment helps treat ulcerative lesions, cryotherapy (ice chips), and keratinocyte growth factor (Palifermin®) have shown some evidence of benefit in the prevention of mucositis
- Systemic opioids may also be needed to adequately control pain and allow improved tolerance of eating.

See UK Oral Mucositis in Cancer Care Group (2015)[2].

Why not screen the population for oral cancer?

Every oral examination by a dental professional must include a check of the soft tissue to exclude any lesion that might be malignant or pre-malignant. So it seems an obviously good idea to reach out to the symptomless population and check them for oral cancer, especially since late presentation is an important problem. Currently, though, the evidence is too limited to support population screening, except in known high-risk populations, e.g. in the Indian subcontinent. This is true even when adjunctive technologies were included like toluidine blue, brush biopsy, or fluorescence imaging. To justify population screening, strict criteria must be met for effectiveness and cost-effectiveness to ensure that the screening does not cause more harm than good, e.g. by detecting false positives, or lesions that would never have progressed or by detecting them still too late to improve mortality or morbidity.

References

1 NICE guideline [NG12] (2015) Suspected cancer: recognition and referral. https://www.nice.org.uk/guidance/ng12
2 UK Oral Mucositis in Cancer Care Group (2015) Mouth care guidance and support in cancer and palliative care. http://www.ukomic.co.uk/new-om-guidelines.html

Saliva

Where does saliva come from?

We produce approximately 1.5 litres of saliva each day from 3 pairs of major glands and accessory minor glands around the mouth, lips, hard and soft palate, buccal mucosa, and circumvallate papilla. At rest, the submandibular gland provides most secretion—a mixture of watery serous and thicker mucous. Minor glands may secrete continuously. (➲ See Table 3.3) When secretion is actively stimulated the parotid provides most volume and the secretion is more watery. Ferguson prefers the term 'oral fluid' to whole saliva because the composition is so variable across time and site[3].

What use is saliva?

Most obvious is the function of saliva in lubricating mastication and swallowing and allowing dissolution of food constituents to provide the sensation of taste. It protects the tissues from drying and allows some mechanical cleansing. But less obviously, there are multiple ways in which saliva is a vital defence for the tissues. It helps maintain the pH of the oral cavity, reduces clotting time of wounds, accelerates wound contraction, reduces aggregation and adherence of bacteria, and has anti-fungal and anti-viral properties. Saliva is also a route for excretion of urea and various drugs (making saliva a convenient means for testing for them).

Constituents of saliva

Strangely, no association has been shown between the ionic composition of saliva and susceptibility to caries or periodontal disease. Key components are:

- Calcium 50% ionic
- Phosphate, mostly in ionic form
- Hydrogen carbonate, an important buffer
- Fluoride, at low levels similar to plasma
- Thiocyanate, lysozyme, and lactoferrin, all antibacterial
- Salivary amylase which begins the digestion of starch.

The pH at rest is 6.5–7.5 but rises as flow increases.

Table 3.3 Salivary glands and their secretions

Name	Type	Resting (%)	Stimulated (%)
Parotid	Mainly serous	Negligible	Predominates
Submandibular	Mixed	Most	30
Sublingual	Mainly mucous	<10	10
Minor	Mucous	<10	10

Circumvallate glands of von Ebner also produce a serous secretion.

Table 3.4 Control of salivary gland secretion

Salivary gland	Sympathetic	Parasympathetic
Parotid	From superior cervical ganglion via external carotid plexus	Inferior salivatory nucleus via glossopharyngeal nerve through tympanic plexus to otic ganglion and auriculo-temporal nerve.
Submandibular and sublingual salivary glands	From superior cervical ganglion via external carotid plexus	Superior salivatory nucleus via chorda tympani branch of facial nerve to submandibular ganglion

How is saliva flow controlled?

Salivation may be provoked by stimuli acting on the salivatory nuclei in the reticular formation (➜ See Table 3.4):

1. Touch, pressure in oral tissues, muscle and joint proprioception
2. Taste
3. Smell
4. Thought

Parasympathetic stimulation increases saliva secretion. Acetylcholine binds to muscarinic receptors on acinar cells, resulting in opening of the potassium channels. Exocytosis releases saliva and chloride ions secreted via a sodium-potassium-chloride transporter. Sympathetic stimulation produces a thick viscous saliva and secretion is reduced to zero during sleep.

How is saliva produced?

The acinus secretes into the intercalated duct which seems to have no specific function. The initial secretion is isotonic with interstitial fluid but with some extra calcium, potassium, and protein. The flow is then to the striated duct (the striated appearance is due to a very infolded basal lamina). Here is the site of major modification of the secretion including active transport of ions, notably the removal of sodium, chloride, and hydrogen carbonate. Various important proteins are added—amylase, lysozyme, lactoferrin, kallikrein, also albumin and urea. Thence saliva flows via excretory ducts to open into the mouth.

The composition of saliva varies with the rate of flow. A fast flow allows less time for re-absorption of hydrogen carbonate so the pH is higher. This helps buffer the effect of plaque acid. Hence the advice to follow a sweet food with cheese or highly flavoured savoury item to keep the flow fast. (➜ See Table 3.5)

Table 3.5 Approximate concentrations mmol/l

	Plasma	Slow flow saliva	Fast flow saliva
Sodium	150	10	80
Chloride	110	10	40
Hydrogen carbonate	25	5	35

Causes of dry mouth

Normal resting flow should be at least 0.25 ml per minute. In older adults resting and stimulated flow seems to be reduced and dry mouth is a common symptom. Xerostomia is the term used for the clinical finding (sign) of dry mouth. There are many potential causes. Note that duct obstruction is not a cause of dry mouth—the other glands compensate.

Direct damage from head and neck radiotherapy
Radiation of head and neck produces changes in salivary gland function, especially parotid. Saliva flow and saliva pH are reduced.

Drug-induced hyposalivation—many drugs can have this side-effect
- **Antihypertensives** e.g. alpha 1 antagonists, alpha 2 agonists, and beta blockers
- **Anticholinergics** e.g. antihistamines, opiates, benzodiazepines, proton-pump inhibitors
- **Antidepressants** (eg selective serotonin re-uptake inhibitors, lithium, tricyclic antidepressants)
- **Diuretics**—because of fluid depletion
- **Cytotoxics**—due to direct damage to actively dividing cells.

Systemic disease
- Sjögren's syndrome—see below
- Pre-existing lymphoma
- Sarcoidosis—chronic granulomatous disease affecting all systems
- Hepatitis C infection
- AIDS—terminal stage of HIV infection
- Graft versus host disease—donor T cells attack the host after a bone marrow transplant, mainly the liver and muco-cutaneous tissues.

Sjögren's syndrome

This is an auto-immune disorder of inflammation of the exocrine glands, which takes two forms:
1. Primary Sjögren's syndrome comprises xerostomia (dry mouth); kerato-conjunctivitis sicca (dry eyes)
2. Secondary Sjögren's syndrome is a triad: xerostomia; kerato-conjunctivitis sicca and a connective tissue disorder usually rheumatoid arthritis

A major complication is the increased risk of developing non-Hodgkin's lymphoma and parotid lymphoma.

What problems arise if saliva production is reduced?

A crucial problem is rampant caries because of reduced buffering capacity and reduced clearance of sugar from the mouth. All possible preventive measures should be applied. There is an increased predisposition to candidiasis and bacterial sialadenitis. Difficulties may also arise with denture retention, chewing, swallowing, and speaking. Management is by stimulation of any residual saliva flow and by saliva substitutes.

How to investigate problems with saliva flow

Sialometry (direct measurement saliva flow) takes 2 forms.

- Unstimulated resting saliva flow is assessed by having the patient collect their saliva in a tube. Normal flow is more than 0.25 ml per minute.
- Stimulated saliva flow is assessed by applying 10% citric acid to the tongue and collecting stimulated saliva directly from the parotid papilla via a suction cup over its opening.

Salivary gland biopsy—usually this is by sampling a few labial glands via a small incision inside the lower lip.

  Sialography is the visualization of the ductal system via injection of a contrast medium into the duct followed by a radiograph.

Can too much saliva be a problem?

Sialorrhoea (excess salivation or hypersecretion) is uncommon.

Causes of true salivary hypersecretion:

1. Local factors such as oral inflammation
2. Menstruation or early pregnancy
3. Medications, e.g. those with cholinergic activity, e.g. pilocarpine, tetrabenazine, clozapine

Causes of difficulty swallowing a normal amount of saliva giving an apparent hypersecretion

- Neuromuscular dysfunction
  - Parkinson's disease
  - Cerebral palsy
  - Learning disability
- Pharyngeal or oesophageal obstruction, e.g. by neoplasm.

Clinical relevance

Management of excess saliva will depend on addressing the cause where possible. Otherwise treatments range from conservative (e.g. exercises, training devices, and biofeedback) to surgical re-routing of the parotid ducts or removal of the submandibular glands but these may have serious adverse effects. More recently ultrasound-guided botulinum toxin injection into the salivary glands has been used. Anticholinergic drugs may help, such as glycopyrronium bromide, benzatropine, or hyoscine hydrobromide.

Reference

[3] Ferguson DB, Shuttleworth A, Whittaker DK. (2006) Oral Bioscience. Sandy : Authors OnLine.

Swallowing

This is a complex sequence of co-ordinated activities which takes place approximately 600 times a day. Only 25% of swallows are part of eating and drinking, most swallowing is to clear unstimulated saliva. The process of swallowing is controlled from a central pattern generator in the medulla oblongata with interconnections to respiratory and cardiovascular centres and the sensory nuclei of V in the pons.

What happens during swallowing?

Swallowing has an oral phase, a pharyngeal phase, and an oesophageal phase as shown in Table 3.6.

Oral phase

In this phase the food is prepared for swallowing. The tongue presses against the hard palate and pushes the bolus posteriorly. The soft palate rests on the posterior part of the tongue.

Pharyngeal phase

In this phase, all the possible alternative exits for the bolus are closed off. The soft palate is elevated and tensed to close off the nasopharynx. The anterior tongue remains pressed against the palate to prevent the food from escaping back into the mouth while the base of the tongue pushes the bolus against the posterior pharyngeal wall. The epiglottis covers the elevated larynx. The upper oesophageal sphincter is relaxed and the palatopharyngeal muscles elevate the oesophagus and positions it beneath the bolus.

Oesophageal phase

The bolus is squeezed into the oesophagus, passing the cricopharyngeal sphincter (which is part of the inferior constrictor muscle). An involuntary, peristaltic wave carries the bolus down the oesophagus.

Clinical application

Impaired swallowing

Normally, swallowing tends to interrupt the expiratory phase of respiration. When the swallow is complete the expiration recommences and will tend to expel any food that remains. In patients with chronic obstructive pulmonary disease (COPD), impaired swallowing is frequently observed. This alteration may be associated with deglutition during inspiration and an increased risk of aspiration of food.

Aspiration pneumonia

Pneumonia arising from aspiration of food, secretions, stomach contents or a foreign body is a complication in dementia, Parkinson's disease, cerebrovascular stroke, multiple sclerosis, and neurological degenerative conditions. There is evidence of an association between oral disease and respiratory disease, especially COPD and pneumonia so additional oral hygiene measures are recommended in susceptible patients to reduce the risk.

Oral cancer

Where oral cancer necessitates resection of the tongue and palatal tissues, there is a reduced propulsive force on the bolus resulting in dysphagia.

Treatments for oral, pharyngeal, or laryngeal cancers by whatever means (surgery, radiotherapy, chemotherapy, or combinations) may give rise to dysphagia as a major side-effect that impacts the quality of life. Dysphagia may continue to worsen for several years after irradiation due to progressive fibrosis and will benefit from specialist rehabilitation.

Cleft palate

For patients with a tissue deficiency of the soft palate, an accurate functional impression of the pharynx is obtained during swallowing movements when constructing speech bulb appliances (obturator).

Choking

This is a medical emergency for which the first aid steps are:
- Encourage the patient to cough. If this does not clear the obstruction then:
- Give 5 back slaps by leaning the patient forward, supporting them with one hand and giving 5 sharp blows with the heel of the other hand between the shoulder blades. If this does not clear the obstruction then:
- Give 5 abdominal thrusts by standing behind the patient, making a fist, placing it between the umbilicus and end of the sternum, placing your other hand over your fist, then pulling sharply inwards and upwards
- Call 999 if the obstruction is not cleared and meanwhile keep alternating 5 back slaps with 5 abdominal thrusts.

Table 3.6 How swallowing takes place

Phases in the normal swallow		
1. Oral preparatory phase		**Muscles involved**
Bolus preparationVoluntary stage V Trigeminal VII Facial IX Glossopharngeal XII Hypoglossal	Soft palate is lowered. Airway open and nasal breathing occurs. Bolus is collected onto dorsum, tongue forms seal against palatal tissue and teeth. Anterior tongue pressed against palatal mucosa.	Palatoglossus, mylohyoid and stylohyoid muscles involved, stylo and hyo-glossus.
2. Oral phase		**Muscles involved**
Voluntary stage	Initiated by the tongue with posterior propulsion of the food bolus. Transition to pharyngeal phase includes elevation of soft palate against the posterior pharyngeal wall which occurs as bolus enters pharynx.	Levator/tensor palatine Superior pharyngeal constrictors contract to help seal nasopharynx
3. Pharyngeal phase		**Muscles involved**
Involuntary and irreversible stage Nerves involved: IX Glossopharyngeal X vagus	Bolus contacts soft palate/ oropharynx. Hyoid, thyroid, and cricoid are raised and move forward by 2 cm. Pharyngeal constrictors contract. Larynx closes at level of epiglottis and vocal cords. Temporary suspension of respiration.	Digastric, geniohyoid and stylohyoid muscles
4. Oesophageal phase		
Involuntary stage Nerves involved: X Vagus	Cricopharyngeal sphincter opens. The bolus is carried into the oesophagus via sequential peristalsis.	Inferior pharyngeal constrictors and oesphageal musculature

Speech

Speech production has three components.

1. **Vocalization** is the production of sound of a particular frequency by expelling air between partly closed vibrating vocal cords. The volume of air expelled determines the loudness of the sound. Length and tension of the cords gives the frequencies.

2. **Phonation** is the process of changing the size and shape of resonating chambers to modify the frequency. These resonating chambers in the head are:
   - Larynx
   - Pharynx—which can be shortened by raising the larynx
   - Nose—which can be closed off by raising the soft palate
   - Mouth—there are two oral resonators:
     — between palate and tongue
     — between lips and teeth, especially the incisors

3. **Articulation** is the pattern of controlled release and stoppage of air flow that gives intelligible speech.
   - For vowels the crucial action is the formation of the oral resonator space.
   - For consonants the crucial action is the controlled release and stoppage of air. This is achieved through the co-ordinated action of lips and tongue against the palate and teeth.

The process is controlled from speech centres in the brain which are mostly on the non-dominant side i.e. on the left in almost all right-handers and the right in around 70% of lefthanders.

The main centres involved are:
- Broca's area for articulation
- Wernicke's area for understanding of speech.

Complex co-ordination of speech and language is achieved through integrated actions between these centres, the auditory cortex (hearing), visual cortex (sight), and hippocampus (memory) all working together.

Important nerves involved in speech are cranial nerves X and VII:
- Vagus (X) is crucial, especially:
  - External laryngeal nerve branch which provides innervation for the crico-thyroid muscle which controls vocal cord length and tension and the crico-pharyneus which acts as a sphincter to keep the oesophagus closed off except during swallowing
  - Recurrent laryngeal nerve supplies the vocalization muscles
- Facial nerve (VII) for facial musculature.

What can go wrong with speech?

→ See Table 3.7. First there are some important terms to know:
- **Dysphasia** is an older term for impaired ability to speak (because dysphasia is so easily confused with dysphagia, i.e. difficulty with swallowing, the term aphasia is preferred).
- **Aphasia**: partial and total language impairment caused by brain injury and stroke
- **Dysarthria**: impaired articulation commonly caused by neuromuscular problems, e.g. Bell's palsy or ill-fitting dentures.

Table 3.7 Mechanism of consonant formation and how changes in certain features of new complete denture may affect them

Name of the sounds	Mechanism	Possible problems
Labial p, b, m	Lip contact	Vertical height Overjet
Labio-dental f, v	Lip to teeth contact	Change in incisor level
Linguodental th	Tip of tongue to upper incisors	Vertical height Overjet
Linguopalatal d, t, l, ch, j	Tongue to hard palate contact	Arch width, palate contour
Linguopalatal h, g, ng	Tongue to soft palate contact	Posterior border of denture is too thick
Nasal m	Air escape from nose, not the mouth	Vertical height Arch width

Clinical application

How to help patients with aphasia?

Aphasia may result from brain injury, brain tumour, neurological disease, dementia, or stroke. Aphasia may be one of the early signs that a stroke is happening. A stroke is a medical emergency and the patient must be taken urgently to an Accident and Emergency centre for assessment, brain imaging, and possible anticoagulants/thrombolysis. Aphasia may affect how someone understands language (receptive aphasia) or their ability to communicate (expressive aphasia).

For patients with aphasia, practical problems arise with history taking, explaining treatment options, and obtaining valid consent. Remember to relate to the patient as an intelligent adult but consider using simpler language and diagrams or pictures as aids.

How might dental procedures affect speech?

Speech sounds may be affected by alterations in the position of the anterior teeth and the shape of the anterior palate.

- The 'th' sound requires the tip of the tongue to momentarily contact the tip of the central incisors.
- The 's' sound requires the tip of the tongue to spread out against the anterior palate but leaving a space for air escape.
- The 'f' and 'v' sounds are formed by the contact of the tips of the upper incisors with the lower lip. Loss of anterior teeth particularly affects these 'f' and 'v' sounds.

In constructing complete dentures, problems may arise with the shape of the anterior palate and the position of the incisors. If the palate is too thin it may allow air to escape during speech and result in a whistling sound. In the same way a large overjet may result in a lisp. A common lisp is caused by mispronunciation of sibilants such as the 's' sound, which may be pronounced as a 'th' sound with the tongue thrusting between the teeth. Any intra-oral device, denture, or appliance may affect speech in the short term but usually adaptation occurs within about a month (Table 3.7).

Cleft palate

Untreated cleft palate is rarely seen now in the UK. The communication through the palate into the nose results in loss of food and liquid into the nose and air escape into the nose gives rise to nasal speech. Ideally, all this is prevented by early surgery at 3 months to repair the palatal defect and allow normal development of speech. The speech and language therapist has a crucial role in the multidisciplinary team caring for cleft patients and speech should be formally assessed at 18 months. A common problem is poor contact between the soft palate and posterior pharynx with incomplete closure of the nasal airway resulting in nasal vocal intonations and further surgery may be needed to correct this.

Bone

Bone structure *86*
Anatomy of bone *88*
Bone turnover *92*
Bone healing *94*
Healing of the extraction socket *98*
Orthodontic tooth movement *100*
Periodontal bone loss in chronic periodontitis *102*
Bisphosphonates *104*
Bone pathology in the elderly *106*
Ageing bone *108*

Bone structure

One of the main properties of bone is that it can maintain rigidity when subjected to muscle action. The stiffness and breaking strain of bone derives from the mineral content, a carbonated hydroxyapatite. For spongy bone, the inorganic component is about 10–20%, with the remainder composed of soft tissue.

Mineral content of bone

Bone undergoes constant turnover, being resorbed by osteoclasts and replaced by osteoblasts. The initial mineralization process of the replaced bone occurs quickly to about two-thirds of the final mineralization content. The remaining third of the mineralization takes years to be completed and finally restored to full mineralization. This slower mineralization process corresponds to a gradual increase in thickness of the mineral plates.

Even within small regions of bone, there is a heterogeneous, mosaic pattern with different degrees of mineralization. This may have an effect on the crack propagation through bone. (➜ See Fig. 4.1)

Clinical relevance

Bisphosphonates inhibit resorption and are used to treat osteoporosis, Paget's disease, bone metastasis, multiple myeloma, and osteogenesis imperfecta. They are released from the bone during resorption and are absorbed into the osteoclast. These drugs inhibit osteoclastic cell function and cause apoptosis; this preventing further resorption. The result for bone structure is to produce a more even pattern of bone mineralization which results in improved physical properties.

The effect of fluoride therapy on bone (at levels higher than 6 mg/day) is to cause an increase in skeletal fragility and fractures. Increased amounts of bone are formed but the deleterious effect of fluoride is caused by its incorporation into the hydroxyapatite crystal and the resultant changes in the size distribution of the mineral particles. GI symptoms are reported as a side-effect of fluoride treatment of osteoporosis. Fluoride therapy (at 2.5–10 mg fluoride/day) is ineffective in treating osteoporosis.

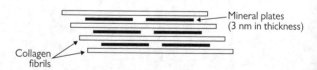

Mineral plates (3 nm in thickness)

Collagen fibrils

Fig. 4.1 Collagen fibrils are interspersed with mineral plates and spaces between the tropocollagen molecules house hydroxyapatite, which reinforces the fibrils and increases their strength.

Matrix content of bone

The matrix of bone is mainly composed of type I collagen, composed of a repeating amino-acid pattern of $(glycine-X-Y)_n$, where X and Y are often proline and hydroxyproline, respectively. This repeating sequence forms a polypeptide chain and three polypeptide chains bind together to form tropocollagen, a coiled helical structure. Osteoblasts deposit the triple-helical collagen molecules in the matrix which self-assemble to form fibrils.

After the formation of tropocollagen, further normal maturation of the collagen involves vitamin C acting as a co-factor in a hydroxylation step. The absence of the hydroxylated residues renders the polypeptide unable to form rigid triple helices and scurvy results.

The toughness of bone depends on the bonds within the tropocollagen molecules and cross linking between adjacent tropocollagen molecules. (See Fig. 4.2)

Clinical relevance

1. Osteogenesis imperfecta: A mutation in the repeating (Gly-X-Y) pattern causes osteogenesis imperfecta, with different effects on the individual's survival depending on the position of the substitution in the molecule.
2. Osteoporosis: Osteoporotic fractures are caused by a reduction in the amount of cortical and cancellous bone. However, the mechanical properties of bone are determined by both the mineral and collagen components and it has been hypothesized that in osteoporosis, changes in the cross-linking of collagen may produce thinner fibrils and bone of reduced strength.
3. Scurvy: If vitamin C is absent from the diet for a period of about 2–3 months then scurvy results. Patients may present with bleeding gums.
4. Ehlers–Danlos syndrome. This is a group of collagen disorders, where the main manifestations are excessive movements of the joints, bruising, and excessive skin extensibility.

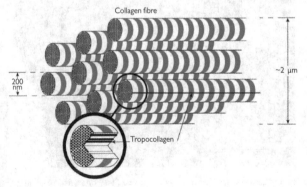

Fig. 4.2 Tropocollagen bound together to form a collagen fibril.

Anatomy of bone

Mature bone is classified as either cortical or cancellous bone.

Gross structure of bone

Cortical bone forms the outer surface layers of bone in the skeleton. It has high density, which provides strength to the bone. Cancellous bone is found mainly at the ends of the long bones (metaphysis and epiphysis) and fills the whole of the interior aspect of the flat bones such as the ribs.

Microscopic structure of bone

Throughout life, bone undergoes a continuous process of resorption and replacement. Bone turnover is necessary for repair of microdamage and for providing adaptation to changes in bone strain. Osteoclasts resorb bone and osteoblasts replace it in a closely coordinated process. In stained decalcified sections of bone, cement lines represent the limit of the osteoclastic resorption. The two cell types have different origins; osteoblasts are derived from mesenchymal stem cells and pericytes, whereas osteoclasts arise from the haemopoietic stem cells.

Osteocyte

These cells lie in lacunae in the calcified matrix of the bone, with fine processes (canaliculi) connecting them to other osteocytes and osteoblasts. These processes terminate in gap junctions. They may provide a local sensory function, initiating resorption of microdamaged bone. (➔ See Fig. 4.3)

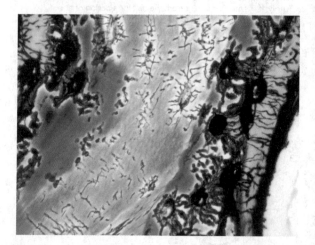

Fig. 4.3 Canaliculi radiate from each of the individual osteocyte lacunae permitting osteocyte communication with each other and with the bone surface osteoblasts/bone-lining cells.

Osteoclast

The osteoclast is a large multinucleated cell. Osteoclasts are mobile cells that have a 'ruffled border' in the region of the cell that lies against the area of bone resorption. The ruffled border of the osteoclast is composed of membrane projections that extend towards the bone surface and increase the available surface area engaged in resorption.

Osteoblast

The osteoblast is connected to adjacent osteoblasts and osteocytes by gap junctions (or intercellular bridges) that allow coordinated roles and actions by groups of cells, e.g. in bone formation. Molecules are able to move between cells through these gap junctions. Osteoblasts are basophilic cells and are found in single layers on the surface of forming bone.

Blood supply to the cortex

The blood supply to the cortex of the long bones is mainly in the centrifugal direction (i.e. towards the outer cortical surface from the more central medullary arteries).

Hypertrophic chondrocytes

During endochondral ossification, fetal bone tissue development and fracture healing, the hypertrophic chondrocyte is the end stage cell of chondrocyte differentiation. These cells are able to undergo further transition at the epiphyseal growth plates to become osteoblasts and osteocytes. The hypertrophic chondrocytes do not undergo programmed cell death, but transform into bone cells.

Thus the mandibular ramus develops from the mandibular condylar cartilage and is therefore chondrocyte-derived, whereas the mandibular body develops through intramembranous bone formation.

Collagen

Collagen is the major protein constituent of bone (95% by weight). It provides flexibility to bone allowing it to bend if suddenly loaded.

Lamellar bone

In lamellar bone, the osteocytes lie in concentric circular or ovoid layers or lamellae. They form cylinders around a central neurovascular channel. These cylinders (or secondary osteons) form the basic unit of organization of cortical bone. Diffusion of nutrients from the central blood vessel throughout the secondary osteon is facilitated by the osteocytic canaliculi. However, the limited diffusion of nutrients affects the maximum diameter of the osteon. (➔ See Fig. 4.4)

Woven bone

Woven bone (➔ See Fig. 4.5) is formed as a result of bone fracture and in initial fetal bone formation. Woven bone is an immature bone where the collagen fibres are arranged in a disordered pattern. Mineralization is rapid. The crystals of mineral in woven bone are smaller than in lamellar bone but have the same plate-like shape.

In Fig. 4.5, new trabeculae of woven bone (thin rods and plates of bone) arising de novo from the marrow and also growing on the surface of a

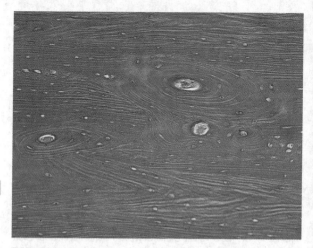

Fig. 4.4 Cortical bone with longitudinal osteons formed of concentric lamellar bone and central Haversian canals containing blood vessels. Between the osteons is interstitial lamellar bone, forming remnants of partially resorbed osteons.

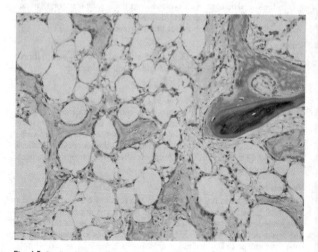

Fig. 4.5 Small trabeculae of woven bone have formed.

pre-existing bone trabeculum (purple-stained bone) are present. These trabeculae are lined by a surface layer of active osteoblasts.

Blood supply to the maxillary bone

In general, the maxilla receives a greater blood supply from the facial artery, through the periosteal vessels, than through the internal maxillary artery, which supplies the endosteal vessels.

Clinical relevance

During maxillary Le Fort 1 osteotomy procedures, ischaemia of bone may cause loss of large parts of the maxilla unless appropriate care is taken to preserve the palatal vasculature. The blood supply of the mobilized Le Fort I maxillary segment is the ascending palatal branch of the facial artery and the anterior branch of the ascending pharyngeal artery. The contralateral facial artery also supplies the maxilla in 50% of cases.

Blood supply to the mandible

The condyle receives a blood supply from mainly endosteal vessels, while the cortical bone in the body of the mandible receives a predominantly periosteal blood supply (mental, submental, and sublingual arteries). The inferior alveolar artery has a main role in the vascular supply to the teeth.

Clinical relevance

Following a diagnosis of oral squamous cell carcinoma, resection of large areas of mandibular bone may be required. This does not usually result in the remaining teeth becoming non-vital due to the extensive, rich collateral blood supply. When the inferior alveolar artery is severed, a collateral blood supply is formed from branches of the facial and lingual arteries.

Perforation of the lingual mandibular cortex during placement of implants in the inter-foraminal region can cause haematoma in the sublingual space. This can be life threatening as the swelling can elevate the tongue and cause respiratory obstruction. The blood vessels affected are the sublingual and submental arteries.

Osteoradionecrosis may follow radiotherapy for malignant disease of the jaws. It is a caused by a reduction in the blood supply to the affected bone resulting in ischaemic necrosis. The mandible is most often affected, with fracture as a late complication. Osteoradionecrosis may be initiated if any flap surgery or tooth extractions are undertaken; therefore patients' dental health must be assessed prior to radiotherapy with regular follow up afterwards.

Bone turnover

Bone is being continually resorbed and deposited throughout the life of an individual. The process is one of harmonious coordination between different cell types with the osteoblast playing the major conducting role. (➲ See Table 4.1 for hormonal influences)

Bone remodelling unit

Osteocytes transmit signals to the osteoblast on the local bone surface to initiate bone resorption. Osteoclasts are stimulated by the osteoblasts to initiate resorption, forming Howship's lacunae. These are seen as resorption craters on the bone surface. On completion of resorption, the osteoclasts undergo apoptosis. Osteoblasts restore the resorbed bone by depositing osteoid, which subsequently mineralizes.

RANKL and OPG

The receptor activator of nuclear factor kappa-B (RANK) ligand is produced by osteoblasts and bone marrow stromal cells and by binding to the RANK receptor on the osteoclast precursor; it causes their differentiation and activation to form osteoclasts.

Osteoprotegerin (OPG) is a member of the TNF receptor superfamily and is produced by osteoblasts, articular chondrocytes, and bone marrow. If OPG is overexpressed in transgenic mice, it causes osteopetrosis as osteoclasts are decreased in number. The main function of OPG is to compete with RANKL for the RANK receptor, thereby preventing osteoclastic proliferation and differentiation. Therefore, OPG and RANKL produce antagonistic effects in bone.

The relative ratio of RANKL and OPG in the bone marrow may be determined by cytokines and hormones, with the result determining whether bone resorption takes place.

Clinical relevance

1. The bone resorption that can occur in metastatic bone tumours is caused by osteoclasts and not by the tumour cells themselves. The bone resorption takes place by osteoclastic activation by the tumour cells and/or the surrounding stromal cells.
2. Denosumab is a monoclonal antibody acting against RANKL.
3. Glucocorticoid-induced osteoporosis occurs through stimulated production of RANKL with simultaneous inhibition of OPG synthesis by osteoblasts.

Table 4.1 Hormonal influence on bone

Hormone causing bone formation	Hormone inhibiting bone resorption	Hormone causing bone resorption
Vitamin D	Calcitonin	Parathyroid hormone

Calcitonin

Calcitonin is produced by the C-cells of the thyroid gland. The effects of calcitonin are to cause:

- An immediate halting of osteoclast activity
- Stimulation 1,25 $(OH)_2$ vitamin D production in the kidney.

However, no bone abnormalities have been reported with excess or diminished production of calcitonin. It may have an important role in maintaining maternal bone mass in pregnancy, in concert with the increased production of 1,25 $(OH)_2$ vitamin D.

Vitamin D

The main effect of 1,25 $(OH)_2$ vitamin D is to increase the absorption of calcium from the GI tract. An inadequate dietary intake of vitamin D will result in a reduced serum concentration of the active vitamin D metabolite, 1,25 $(OH)_2$ vitamin D.

Therefore the effects of a reduced serum 1,25 (OH)2 vitamin D is to cause

1. Hyperparathyroidism
2. Osteomalacia

Parathyroid hormone

When the serum concentration of Ca^{2+} is reduced, receptors in the parathyroid gland detect this and the gland secretes parathyroid hormone. This hormone acts on the bone (stimulating bone resorption) and the kidney (stimulating synthesis of 1,25$(OH)_2$ vitamin D which increases the intestinal absorption of calcium). In a negative feedback loop, 1,25$(OH)_2$ vitamin D reduces transcription and secretion of parathyroid hormone.

Clinical relevance

1,25$(OH)_2$ vitamin D (or precursor) may be used to treat patients with secondary hyperparathyroidism resulting from chronic kidney disease, with the aim of reducing the serum parathyroid hormone concentration.

Cementocyte

Bone undergoes continuous turnover with osteocytes playing a central role, whereas cementum has no turnover and cementocytes do not play any role in regulating systemic mineral metabolism. Cementum is a bone-like mineralized tissue that covers the root dentine. In the apical region, the cementum contains embedded cementocytes and is therefore called cellular cementum. Cementocytes resemble osteocytes in that they are buried in a calcified matrix and form canalicular connections with each other. The higher OPG/RANKL ratio in cementocytes may offer protection from osteoclastic resorption of cementum under normal conditions.

Bone healing

Fracture healing of the long bones

Following fracture of a long bone a blood clot forms between the bone ends. An inflammatory phase occurs in the first week with the appearance of macrophages and the release of growth factors. The fracture haematoma and adjacent bone marrow stimulate periosteal cell proliferation. This is followed by replacement of the blood clot with granulation tissue. Bone resorption occurs. Undifferentiated mesenchymal cells populate the area and these divide and differentiate into either chondrocytes or osteoblasts with matrix formation, forming a soft callus. The growth factors released by the periosteum are important in stimulating chondrogenesis. (→ See Figs 4.6 and 4.7)

The fracture matrix

Secretion of collagen types I and III is associated with the osteoblast lineage and formation of woven bone, whereas collagen type II and X are present in the cartilaginous callus.

Bone formation

The series of cellular histological changes occurring during healing of long bone fractures resembles that which takes place during bone development in the embryo. Bone forms during development either as a result of intramembranous ossification or through endochondral ossification. Intramembranous bone forms at the periosteal surface whereas endochondral ossification requires a process of cartilage synthesis followed by its replacement by bone.

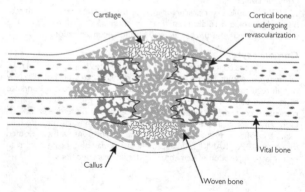

Fig. 4.6. Fracture repair of a long bone.

Maturation of the newly calcified tissue

Fracture healing of long bones involves both intramembranous and endochondral ossification. The newly formed calcified tissue stabilizes the two bone ends, and there is a gradual increase in the strength of the callus with time. There is a remodelling period in which the woven bone and calcified cartilage of the hard callus is replaced by a lamellar type of bone.

Mesenchymal stem cells (MSC) are critical to the success of fracture healing
These cells:
- Are normally present in the bone marrow, periosteum and endosteum
- Migrate to the site of injury due to chemokines (e.g. stromal cell-derived factor, SDF-1) released following the resulting tissue hypoxia
- MSC inhibit fibrosis and differentiate into osteoblasts and chondrocytes.

Administering MSC to experimental animals with bone fractures has a moderately beneficial effect. Systemically administered MSC have proved effective when concentrated populations are used to promote bone healing.

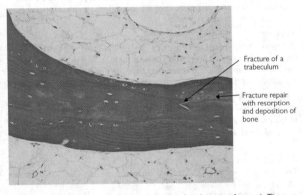

Fracture of a trabeculum

Fracture repair with resorption and deposition of bone

Fig. 4.7 Repair of fracture of a single bone trabeculum (i.e. microfracture). The outline of the original, pre-fracture bone trabecula is defined by the cement line. There is a crack in the bone across the trabeculum with evidence of surface bone resorption at the site of this microfracture and osteocyte necrosis (i.e. empty osteocytic lacunae within the confines of the cement lines—i.e. the original bone trabecula). There is apposition of viable new bone on the trabecular surface bridging, and healing, the microfracture. In miniature, this figure shows essentially similar features of the same cycle of bone resorption and deposition as occurs in a fracture of the whole bone.

Clinical relevance

The amount of movement between the fractured bone ends determines whether healing occurs through bone union (direct healing) or by bone replacement of cartilage (indirect healing).

Bone grafts

When reconstruction of the jaws occurs after surgery to remove cancer or other pathology, a bone graft may be used. The jaw bones undergo continuous reduction in height following extraction of the teeth, therefore bone grafts may be used in this situation to provide a sufficient volume of bone to allow placement of titanium implants.

Bone grafts can be divided into two broad groups of materials.

- An osteoinductive material stimulates the recruitment of osteoprogenitor cells and their differentiation to form new bone. This can occur following implantation of an osteoinductive material in muscle.
- An osteoconductive material allows bone to form on its surface. Bone grows on the bioinert surface of titanium implants, producing a stable union. There is no cartilaginous phase, but a direct union is formed; a process called osseointegration.

Autograft

These are grafts taken from another site of the same individual. Due to their rapid healing and stimulation of new bone, autografts are considered the ideal graft material. However, they have the disadvantage of donor site morbidity and the amount of graft bone that can be harvested is limited.

Allograft (e.g. demineralized freeze-dried bone)

This is bone that has been collected from another individual and sterilized to remove any contaminating organisms. There is a risk of rejection of the donated tissue, but this is minimized by processing techniques that remove the cells.

Graft substitutes

These include materials such as hydroxyapatite, Bio-Oss®, β-tricalcium phosphate, and bioactive glass. (➔ See Fig. 4.8)

- Hydroxyapatite grafts appear as densely radiopaque materials on radiographs and are therefore easily distinguished from the surrounding bone. It is non-resorbable.
- Bio-Oss® is an anorganic bovine bone material. It resorbs very slowly.
- β-tricalcium phosphate grafts resorb completely and are replaced by bone. It has osteoconductive properties.
- Bioactive glass. These materials bond to bone and the products of the graft dissolution stimulate new bone formation.

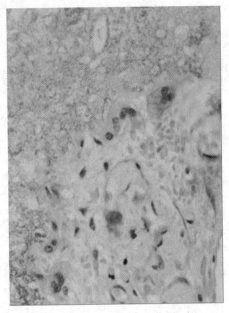

Fig. 4.8 Resorption of a graft substitute material by osteoclast-like cells.

Healing of the extraction socket

The main distinguishing feature between the healing of long bone fractures and extraction sockets is the absence of cartilage in the latter.

The process involves several histological stages:

1. A blood clot is formed. Inflammatory cells (neutrophils) are evident in the superficial part of the clot. In the early stages, the residual fibres of the periodontal ligament are present.
2. Fibroblasts and blood vessels invade the blood clot with formation of granulation tissue. Osteoclasts resorb the bone lining the extraction socket.
3. Woven bone is deposited in the fibrous tissue matrix. This bone forms adjacent to blood vessels in the socket.
4. The woven bone is replaced by lamellar bone. Primary osteons are seen. The socket is covered with epithelium. The surface of the socket is covered by a hard tissue layer of lamellar and woven bone on which lies a periosteum.

The origin of the cells forming the woven bone is controversial. Likely candidates include the residual periodontal ligament, bone marrow cells and/or cells surrounding the blood vessels (pericytes).

Clinical implications

The residual bone following a tooth extraction continues to resorb, with the major part of the resorption occurring in the first six months after extraction. The amount of jaw bone resorption varies widely between individuals and is impossible to predict.

Alveolar osteitis ('dry socket')

This is a painful condition that usually is evident two or three days after the tooth extraction. There is usually an empty extraction socket, with disintegration of the blood clot within the socket. It affects about 3% of people having otherwise uneventful tooth extraction, but the incidence is increased approximately tenfold in those who have received a surgical extraction for the removal of impacted third molars.

Pathogenesis

The primary event is the disintegration of the blood clot by fibrinolytic activity of either endogenous or bacterial origin.

Antiseptic mouthrinses (such as chlorhexidine) reduce the incidence of alveolar osteitis, which implies a bacterial aetiology. *Streptococcus mutans*, *Actinomyces viscosus*, and anaerobic organisms have been proposed as the causative organisms. The anaerobic bacterial organism *Treponema denticola* is a pathogen in periodontal disease and its fibrinolytic activity may be responsible for removing the blood clot. Previous infection of the surgical site (such as pericoronitis) increases the risk of alveolar osteitis.

Alternative theories involve excessive trauma causing inflammation of the bone surrounding the socket, and the release of activators of fibrinolytic activity in the blood clot.

Summary of predisposing conditions

Alveolar osteitis occurs more frequently in those individuals with the following pre-disposing conditions:

• A difficult traumatic extraction
• Smoking tobacco (with nicotine acting as a vasoconstrictor)
• Women taking oral contraceptives
• Patients with pre-existing pericoronitis

Prevention of alveolar osteitis

Chlorhexidine rinses, administered before surgery, have been shown to be useful in reducing the incidence of alveolar osteitis. Chlorhexidine is an antiseptic reagent.

Preoperative antibiotics, such as metronidazole, topical tetracycline, or topically applied clindamycin, have also been shown to be effective, but giving pre-operative antibiotics is controversial as there may be an increased risk of developing resistant bacterial organisms and hypersensitivity reactions.

Using the minimum of surgical trauma during tooth extraction is important in reducing the incidence of alveolar osteitis. There is no evidence to show that placing a post-operative dressing is effective in prevention.

Some studies have shown that a previous history of alveolar osteitis may increase a patient's risk of future episodes. This may indicate a genetic predisposition of these patients to this condition.

Treatment of alveolar osteitis

Gentle irrigation of the socket with warm saline solution is recommended with application of an iodoform ribbon gauze dressing coated with a paste of eugenol and zinc oxide. The dressing should be changed every 2–3 days.

Healing of the affected socket can be prolonged. About half of patients with alveolar osteitis require four or more postoperative visits to the clinic to change the dressing until the symptoms finally resolve[1].

Reference

[1] Osborn TP, Frederickson G Jr, Small IA, Torgerson TS. (1985) A prospective study of complications related to mandibular third molar surgery. *J Oral Maxillofac Surg.*; **43**:767–9.

Orthodontic tooth movement

Removable orthodontic appliances incorporate springs which are able to apply a continuous force to the clinical crown and tip teeth. The centre of rotation is in the apical third of the root. If the tooth is moved away from the midline, there is a pressure zone on the distal surface of the tooth and a tension zone on the mesial surface. The activity of the osteoclasts in the pressure zone and the osteoblasts in the tension zone is balanced to maintain the width of the periodontal ligament.

Clinical observations

When the clinician activates the spring on an orthodontic appliance to initiate tooth movement, there is a delay while cell recruitment occurs to the region. Bone turnover commences, and tooth movement occurs until the spring becomes deactivated. Bone resorption occurs adjacent to the pressure zone of the periodontal ligament, with bone deposition on the tension side. Ideally, light forces should be used clinically.

Bone formation at the palatal suture

In orthodontic appliances for applying rapid maxillary expansion, tension forces are generated at the midline palatal suture. Bone is deposited in this region.

The pressure zone

The alveolar bone surface undergoing pressure undergoes resorption, with formation of a hyalinized zone in the adjacent periodontal ligament. The hyalinized zone is a cell-free area with a ground glass histological appearance. Activation of bone resorption requires a period of several days before it starts. In the hyalinization zone, the alveolar bone is undermined by osteoclasts from surrounding bone rather than resorption of bone adjacent to the periodontal ligament. The mechanical stimulus alters the bone strain which activates remodelling resulting in bone resorption. Some micro-damage in the periodontal ligament is also observed and the resulting sterile inflammation and tissue ischaemia may also stimulate osteoclastic bone resorption. Heavy orthodontic forces increase the amount of hyalinization and undermining bone resorption.

The tension zone

Bone resorption also occurs on the tension side. It is followed by inhibition of further resorption and a phase of deposition of bone. Bone deposition results from the mechanical bending of the bone. Continuous light forces of 25–50 g will cause tooth movement, without causing root resorption.

Root resorption in fixed orthodontic treatment

Root resorption occurs more frequently with fixed appliance than removable appliance therapy. Where the roots are thin and short, there is an increased risk of more severe root resorption. A typical course of orthodontic treatment results in about 1–2 mm of apical root loss, which is not clinically significant. Resorption on the lateral surfaces of teeth is also possible, but this is not usually visible on 2-D radiographic images unless it is severe.

Management of alveolar clefts

The primary anomaly in cleft lip and palate is the deficiency of bone and soft tissue in this region resulting from a failure in development. The bone grafting techniques and timing for the optimal aesthetic and functional result are not universally agreed. Typically, lip closure occurs at 3–6 months of age with palatal closure at 9–12 months.

In the UK, secondary maxillary bone grafting and surgical repair occur at about 8–11 years of age, which allows the canine to erupt into the grafted zone. The surgery also aims to provide stability of the premaxilla, improved occlusion, and continuity of the dental arches.

The most common donor site is the iliac crest, but this is prone to rapid resorption in the first year after placement. If there is failure of eruption of the canine tooth into the graft, then resorption of the graft is greater than if the canine does erupt into the graft[2].

Other complications include graft dehiscence and infection.

Surgical exposure of impacted canines

Impacted maxillary canines are often exposed surgically and orthodontically moved into the line of the dental arch. Trauma to the periodontal ligament during surgery can result in ankylosis of the canine (occurring as frequently as 14.5% of cases). This is associated with replacement resorption of the root.

Autotransplantation of teeth with complete roots has a success rate of about 70% over 5 years. Placing the teeth in light occlusal contact is beneficial in preventing ankylosis.

Distraction osteogenesis

This surgical technique is used to correct developmental defects of the facial region, e.g. cleft lip and palate, mandibular and mid-face hypoplasia and asymmetry. In this technique the bone is cut and the two bone fragments slowly pulled apart to induce bone formation in the gap. This versatile technique produces more stable results than traditional grafting.

Reference

2 Zhang W, Shen G, Wang X, Yu H, Fan L. (2012) Evaluation of alveolar bone grafting using limited cone beam computed tomography. *Oral Surg Oral Med Oral Pathol Oral Radiol.* **113**:542–8.

Periodontal bone loss in chronic periodontitis

Loss of bone from around the teeth is commonly caused by chronic periodontitis, which leads to a progressive destruction of the periodontal attachment. The amount of attachment loss is calculated by adding the amount of tissue loss due to gingival recession to the depth of the gingival pocket.

Chronic periodontitis is initiated by bacterial plaque. The host response is the release of host proinflammatory cytokines and matrix metalloproteinases that causes destruction of the connective tissue in a susceptible individual. This chronic inflammation results in an increase in the RANKL/OPG ratio, which stimulates the differentiation of osteoclasts and bone resorption. OPG and RANKL are competitive for the RANK binding site on the osteoclast precursor cell. OPG prevents the formation of osteoclasts whereas RANKL stimulates osteoclast differentiation and bone resorption.

If plaque is not removed and allowed to mature on the tooth, the early signs of gingivitis begin to be seen at about day 3. If the plaque is left undisturbed for longer, there is a change in plaque composition after about a week or so. The plaque consists mainly of gram-positive facultative bacteria at an early stage, but this later changes to a predominantly gram-negative, anaerobic flora containing, e.g. *Bacteroides forsythus* or *Porphyromonas gingivalis*.

Epidemiology

Periodontal bone loss increases with age due to the accumulated episodes of disease experienced over the years.

The severity of chronic periodontitis may be increased in those with:
• Poorly controlled diabetes mellitus
• Smoking habits
• Stress.

Local risk factors for chronic periodontitis include enamel pearls, overhanging restorations, tooth furcations etc.

Assessment of periodontal bone loss

Assessment of alveolar bone loss is by visual examination, clinical probing, and radiographs.

Visual examination

There may be few signs of gingival inflammation, especially if the patient is maintaining their oral hygiene. However, in severe disease the patient may complain of mobile teeth and migration of the anterior teeth.

Clinical probing

Periodontal pockets are present with loss of clinical attachment. Bleeding may be apparent from the gingival pocket following gentle probing.

Radiographic examination

In health, the crest of the alveolar bone is situated 2 mm from the cemento-enamel junction. Chronic periodontitis is associated with alveolar bone loss that is seen on bitewing radiography.

Classification of chronic periodontitis

Chronic periodontitis can be classified as either:

- Localized involving 30% of sites or fewer
- Generalized involving more than 30% of sites.

The severity of chronic periodontitis is classified using attachment loss, and is classified as slight with 1–2 mm loss, moderate involving 3–4 mm loss, or severe >5 mm.

The morphology of the periodontal defect

The response to treatment of periodontal defects depends on their morphology with 3-walled defects healing in a more predictable manner than 1 or 2-walled defects. The poorer prognosis may relate to the distance that cells must migrate if they are to successfully populate the larger defects. (➲ See Fig. 4.9)

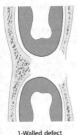 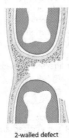 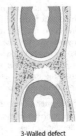

1-Walled defect   2-walled defect   3-Walled defect

Fig. 4.9 Guided tissue regeneration is a barrier technique that allows fibroblasts from the remaining periodontal ligament to populate the defect and create a new periodontal attachment. The apical migration of gingival epithelium and population of the defect with gingival connective tissue is prevented.

Bisphosphonates

These drugs inhibit osteoclastic resorption of bone but use of the more potent intravenous agents or prolonged oral use (after 2 years) have the side-effect of causing osteonecrosis of the jaw. Their main effect is to inhibit osteoclasts, and it is therefore used to prevent fractures in osteoporosis, and treat Paget's disease and malignancies metastatic to bone.

Medication-related osteonecrosis of the jaws (MRONJ)

Typically, osteonecrosis becomes evident following tooth extraction with exposure of the jaw bone and failure of healing of the socket. Persisting infection may cause swelling and abscess formation and altered sensation (hypoesthesia or paraesthesia) of the lips. With more extensive and severe involvement of the jaws, chronic osteomyelitis is seen with the radiographic appearance of a periosteal reaction and sequestra formation.

The jaws are affected because of their high bone turnover, resulting in concentration of bisphosphonate as it binds to the hydroxyapatite. This binding of the bisphosphonate occurs at neutral pH, but the effect of infection may be to cause acidification of the tissues and release of the hydroxyapatite locally, causing a cytotoxic effect. Bisphosphonates are known to have an anti-angiogenic effect.

The mandible is more often affected by medication-related osteonecrosis than the maxilla. This may relate to differences in the blood supply of the mandible and maxilla.

Radiographic findings

On panoramic radiographs, the poorly healed extraction socket can be identified. The appearance of the affected area can be lytic, sclerotic, or a mixture of both types. Sclerosis may cause an increased thickness of the lamina dura of any adjacent teeth accompanied by thickening of the mandibular canal.

Prevention

With liaison between the dentist and the medical practitioner, patients should be rendered dentally fit prior to commencing bisphosphonate therapy. At this stage, the possibility of future extractions should be assessed, inadequate restorations replaced, and oral hygiene measures instituted. When the patient, who is at risk of developing osteonecrosis, has commenced treatment with bisphosphonates, they should receive recalls every 2–3 months to monitor their dental health. Later, they should receive endodontic treatment in preference to tooth extraction.

There is no evidence that stopping bisphosphonate therapy prior to a dental procedure will reduce the risk of osteonecrosis.

Treatment

Osteonecrosis is slow to heal. The treatment is usually conservative with the use of antiseptic rinses and systemic antibiotics to control the infection. Surgery should be limited to local debridement to remove easily removed bone sequestra. The lifting of extensive flaps will only exacerbate and prolong the healing process.

Other treatments have been recommended:

1. Hyperbaric oxygen: The increased oxygenation of the tissues may increase the concentration of free radicals provided by macrophages at the healing site. Hyperbaric oxygen may be useful in the treatment of those patients with severe medication-related osteonecrosis. It may help to relieve the pain symptoms in this group.

However, the evidence supporting the use of hyperbaric oxygen in osteonecrosis is weak. In a randomized controlled trial of hyperbaric oxygen treatment by Freiberger et al (2012), 46 patients were followed for two years. No statistically significant differences in the complete gingival coverage were seen between the control and treatment groups. The study was under-powered[3].

A Cochrane Review by Rollason et al (2016) found studies supporting the use of hyperbaric oxygen in treating MRONJ but these studies provided a poor quality of evidence[4].

2. Ozone therapy has been recommended for the treatment of medication-related osteonecrosis of the jaw, but the evidence supporting its use is weak. It has been reported anecdotally to improve symptoms.

MRONJ was first identified as a side-effect of bisphosphonates, but more recently other drugs have been implicated. These are other antiresorptives, e.g. denosumab, and some antiangiogenic drugs.

References

[3] Freiberger JJ, Padilla-Burgos R, McGraw T, Suliman HB, Kraft KH, Stolp BW, Moon RE, Piantadosi CA. (2012) What is the role of hyperbaric oxygen in the management of bisphosphonate-related osteonecrosis of the jaw: a randomized controlled trial of hyperbaric oxygen as an adjunct to surgery and antibiotics. *J Oral Maxillofac Surg* **70**:1573–83.

[4] Rollason V, Laverrière A, MacDonald LCI, Walsh T, Tramèr MR, Vogt-Ferrier NB. Interventions for treating bisphosphonate-related osteonecrosis of the jaw (BRONJ). *Cochrane Database of Systematic Reviews* 2016, Issue 2. Art. No.: CD008455.

Bone pathology in the elderly

Post-menopausal osteoporosis

Women frequently develop bone resorption as a result of the reduction in serum oestrogen following the menopause. In the jaws, radiographs show a sparse trabecular pattern and thinning of the mandibular cortex. There are serious general medical complications such as an increasing incidence of fractures of the hip, wrist, and vertebrae as the patients get older.

Diagnosing post-menopausal osteoporosis

Using selected clinical information and a measurement of mandibular cortical width on panoramic radiographs, an index can be produced which has value in predicting hip fracture[5].

Osteoporotic patients have fewer teeth

In a large multi-centre study funded by a project grant from the European Commission FP5 'Quality of life and management of living resources', it was shown that there was a significant association between osteoporosis at the hip or spine and tooth loss. After adjusting for age and smoking, osteoporotic patients had about one fewer tooth[6].

Oral cancer

The incidence of oral cancer rises steeply from the age of about 40 years, with men more frequently affected than women. About three-quarters of deaths from oral cancer occur in those aged 60 years and over.

The main risk factors for oral cancer are excessive consumption of alcohol (especially of spirits), tobacco, and betel nut. The pooled effect of excessive consumption of alcohol and smoking is synergistic. Human papilloma virus (HPV) is also an important aetiological agent in the onset of HPV-positive oropharyngeal squamous cell carcinoma. HPV-positive oropharyngeal tumours have higher radio-sensitivity and improved survival over HPV-negative oropharyngeal cancer patients.

Bone invasion in oral squamous cell carcinoma

When oral squamous cell carcinoma has advanced to invade mandibular bone, the prognosis is much reduced. Histologically, three patterns have been described:

- An infiltrative pattern (characterized by projections of tumour cells into the bone along an irregular front)
- Erosive pattern (where there is a distinct demarcation between the tumour and the surrounding bone)
- Mixed type showing features of both erosive and infiltrative pattern.

The oral squamous cell carcinoma usually invades the adjacent mandible at the reflection of the attached gingiva and the lingual mucosa.

Mechanism of bone resorption in oral cancer

It is now generally accepted that the cancer cells do not directly resorb bone, but that this is mediated by osteoclasts. The RANKL/RANK system is extremely important in inducing differentiation of osteoclasts. RANKL is produced by cancer stromal cells following the stimulation from interleukin-6 and parathyroid hormone-related protein released by the cancer cells.

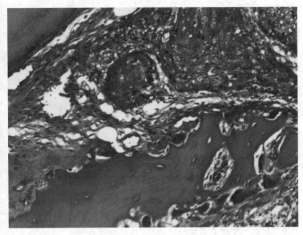

Fig. 4.10 A poorly differentiated squamous cell carcinoma metastatic to bone. The presence of the metastasis has stimulated bone resorption via the many multi-nucleated osteoclasts that are present on the bone surface.

There is a simultaneous reduction in the expression of osteoprotegerin in the stromal cells which also tends to encourage osteoclastogenesis. The osteoclasts release growth factors which stimulate tumour cell proliferation.

The increased release of cytokines by the stromal cells may be responsible for the infiltrative pattern of bone invasion observed histologically. (➔ See Fig. 4.10)

References

5 Horner K, Allen P, Graham J, Jacobs R, Boonen S, Pavitt S, Nackaerts O, Marjanovic E, Adams JE, Karayianni K, Lindh C, van der Stelt P, Devlin H. (2010) The relationship between the OSTEODENT index and hip fracture risk assessment using FRAX. Oral Surg Oral Med Oral Pathol Oral Radiol Endod. **110**:243–9.

6 Nicopoulou-Karayianni K1, Tzoutzoukos P, Mitsea A, Karayiannis A, Tsiklakis K, Jacobs R, Lindh C, van der Stelt P, Allen P, Graham J, Horner K, Devlin H, Pavitt S, Yuan J. (2009) Tooth loss and osteoporosis: the OSTEODENT Study. *J Clin Periodontol*. **36**:190–7.

Ageing bone

Throughout maturity, bone formation and resorption are balanced. However, in old age, bone resorption exceeds bone deposition. Bone turnover is necessary to repair microdamage and to meet the changing functional demands of the skeleton.

There are changes in cortical bone which takes place with ageing and which can be used to indicate the approximate age of an individual. This could be important in the forensic identification of murder victims and in archaeological examinations.

Age changes in bone structure

The main effect of age is to cause a reduction in peak bone mass in the body from about the age of 30 years, with an acceleration in women around the peri-menopausal period. The menopausal bone loss is associated with an irreversible perforation of the trabecular plates, caused by osteoclastic activity. Older bone is preferentially resorbed. This may be due to its different structure, resulting from increased carbonate and hydroxyl substitution in the bone mineral.

Cortical bone changes with age

As individuals become older, the cortical bone becomes more porous with osteoclastic resorption of the cortical bone causing an increased number of fragmented osteons. These changes are seen on histological sections of the long bone.

Cortical resorption also takes place at the endosteal surface of the mandible, causing thinning of the cortical layer. This can be observed as a thinning of the inferior mandibular cortex. Excessive thinning of the mandibular cortex is found in female patients with osteoporosis[8].

Trabecular bone changes with age

There is a loss of trabecular bone with age, caused by thinning and perforation of the trabeculae by osteoclastic resorption. In general, the removal of trabeculae and their increased separation has a more significant influence than trabecular thinning in causing a deterioration of the mechanical properties of bone.

How does ageing affect bone cells

Mesenchymal stem cells

Mesenchymal stem cells are capable of differentiating into different tissues such as bone cells, fibroblasts, and cells of cartilage, muscle, and adipose tissue. However, with age they lose the potential to proliferate and differentiate and become senescent. As they age, mesenchymal stem cells tend to favour adipogenic differentiation rather than osteogenic differentiation.

Osteocytes

Young osteocytes secrete a matrix which mineralizes, except for a thin osteoid layer (or pericellular sheath) remaining around the cells. Older osteocytes may resorb surrounding bone before undergoing apoptosis or programmed cell death. Osteocyte apoptosis increases with age.

Osteoclasts

Human marrow cells have been shown in vitro to have an increased osteo-clastogenic potential and expression of receptor activator of NF-κB ligand (RANKL) with age. There may be an increased differentiation of osteoclasts from mesenchymal stem cells with age.

Osteoblasts

A result of ageing is that the amount of bone deposited by osteoblasts at each remodelling cycle is reduced. This could be due to a decreased recruit-ment of osteoblast precursors to the bone deposition site or a reduced lifespan of osteoblasts.

The lifespan of a cell is limited to a certain number of replications which decreases with age. With each cell division, the telomere at the end of the chromosome decreases in length, finally resulting in cell apoptosis. Telomerase maintains the length of the telomeres and is very active in cells with unlimited replicative ability, e.g. mesenchymal stem cells.

Mesenchymal stem cells can differentiate into multiple cell types, but they are only present in small numbers in adult bone marrow. This requires them to be isolated and their numbers expanded in vitro before they can be reintroduced back into the patient. Unfortunately, mesenchymal stem cells

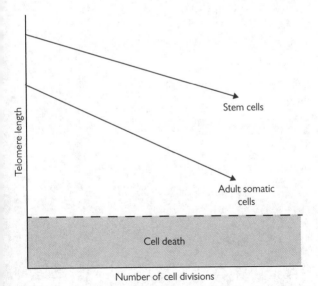

Fig. 4.11 Telomerase activity is quiescent in most adult cells, except adult stem cells, and is an indicator of biological ageing.

undergo loss of telomere length during the expansion process resulting in cells that have short telomeres and severely compromised replicative ability. The age of the donor also has a significant effect on the replicative ability of the donated mesenchymal stem cells. (➜ See Fig. 4.11)

Reference

[8] Roberts M, Yuan J, Graham J, Jacobs R, Devlin H. (2011) Changes in mandibular cortical width measurements with age in men and women. *Osteoporos Int* **22**:1915–25.

Chapter 5

Liver

Structure of the liver 112
Functions of the liver 114
Drugs and the liver 116
Alcohol and the dental patient 120
Liver disease 122
Hepatitis 124
Tests for liver function 128
Management of dental care in patients with impaired liver
    function 130

Structure of the liver

The liver is the largest organ at 1–1.5 kg and it has a key role in many body functions. It fortunately has the ability to regenerate quickly if some liver tissue is damaged. It is said that 80% of the liver capacity is excess.

Anatomy of the liver

- Located in the right upper quadrant of the abdomen
- The liver has a covering of peritoneum
- There are 4 anatomical lobes (right, left, caudate, quadrate) each with 4 segments
- Afferent blood supply is by the hepatic artery from the coeliac axis
- Portal vein brings nutrient rich blood from the gut (superior mesenteric vein and splenic vein)
- Efferent blood supply is by the hepatic vein to inferior vena cava.

The functional unit of the liver is the lobule, 1–2 mm across, each of these hexagonal collections of cells consists of hepatocytes radiating around a central vein which feeds ultimately into the hepatic vein. Single cell layers of hepatocytes drain into blind-ended canaliculi which ultimately drain into the bile duct. At each of the 6 corners of the lobule is a triad of vessels comprising a branch of bile duct, portal vein, and hepatic artery.(➲ See Figs 5.1 and 5.2)

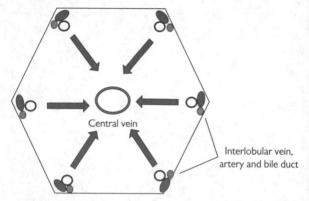

Central vein

Interlobular vein, artery and bile duct

Fig. 5.1 A liver lobule with blood flowing through sinusoids to the central vein.

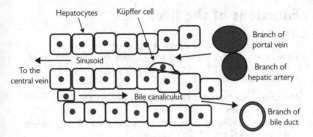

Fig. 5.2 Blood flowing through sinusoids to the central vein and bile collecting in bile canaliculi.

Functions of the liver

The three major functions of the liver are:
1. Metabolism of nutrients and toxins absorbed from intestines
2. Exocrine function producing bile which helps carry away waste and break down fats in the small intestine during digestion
3. Synthesis of many crucial products

Metabolism of nutrients and toxins absorbed from intestines

- All the blood from the stomach and intestines passes first to the liver and then slowly through the hepatic lobules.
- Amino acids, fatty acids, and glucose are removed from the blood for processing or storage.
- Glycogen is formed and stored, then released under hormonal control.
- A key process is deamination in which toxic ammonia is removed from amino acids via the urea cycle and converted to urea which is excreted in the urine. The process of transamination allows any needed amino acids to be constructed by the liver from dietary protein, glucose, and proteins undergoing turnover.
- Fatty acids are oxidized, triglycerides and cholesterol are synthesized
- Bile salts are metabolized. They are required for fat-soluble vitamins to be absorbed.
- Copper and iron are stored in the liver.
- Vitamins A, D, K, and B^{12} are stored in the liver.
- Vitamin K is used in production of prothrombin (Factor VII).
- 25-hydroxylation of Vitamin D takes place in liver.
- Some hormones are inactivated, e.g. oestrogens and other steroids are conjugated to glucuronic acid, insulin, glucagon, and growth hormone are degraded mainly by the liver and the kidneys.
- Some drugs are detoxified.
- Phagocytic (Kupffer) cells in the liver remove and destroy bacteria that have evaded other defences of the digestive tract and entered hepatic portal circulation. Some old erythrocytes or red blood cells (RBCs) are also destroyed here (most in the spleen).

Exocrine function

Bile consists of a sodium bicarbonate solution containing:
- Bile salts which emulsify and aid absorption of lipids. Bile salts are almost completely reabsorbed from the small intestine, entering the entero-hepatic circulation to be recycled with very little escaping into the faeces and contributing to its colour.
- Bile pigments (chiefly bilirubin) are formed in the reticuloendothelial system, e.g. spleen by the breakdown of RBCs. Gut bacteria convert bilirubin to urobilinogen, some of which is excreted in faeces, some of which is reabsorbed for reuse in bile or excreted via the kidneys. In jaundice, bilirubin escapes into the circulation and shows as a yellow colouration in the sclera and skin.

- Cholesterol and lecithin.

Cholesterol has complex functions as the basis for steroid hormones, vitamin D and plasma membranes. Excess is excreted in bile and lecithin helps it dissolve.

Around 250–1,000 ml of bile is produced daily and stored in the gallbladder. Fat entering the duodenum stimulates the intestinal mucosa to release cholecystokinin which causes the gallbladder to contract, releasing bile into the small intestine.

Synthesis

The liver has a crucial role in producing some key proteins.

a. Many globulins of the clotting cascade:
  - Clotting factors I (fibrinogen), II, V, VII, IX, X, XI, XII, XIII
  - Prothrombin

The half-life of many of these proteins is short (hours) so an early sign of problems with liver function will show in blood clotting.

b. Antibodies or immunoglobins (gamma globulin, IgG, IgE, IgA, IgD, IgM).

c. Plasma albumin (large colloidal protein molecules), the most common protein in the blood on which depends the oncotic pressure of blood. It retains fluid in the circulation and if albumin is depleted then fluid leaves the circulation and tissue oedema results.

Drugs and the liver

The liver has a crucial role in handling drugs.
1. It produces plasma proteins which are involved in transport or binding of drugs.
2. It is the major site for metabolizing drugs.
3. The liver excretes some drug products into the bile.

Drugs and plasma proteins

The main effect of plasma proteins on drugs is in their transport and distribution. Key plasma proteins in this context are albumin, acid-glycoprotein, and beta-globulin. Circulating drugs may bind to plasma proteins, but this binding is rapidly reversible and non-specific. Such bound drug acts as a reservoir of the drug, but only the free, unbound drug will have a therapeutic effect.

There are several important implications of plasma protein binding of drugs.

- If plasma proteins levels are low then the same drug dosage will produce a greater effect than expected. This may occur in old age, malnutrition, liver failure (due to less plasma protein produced), or kidney failure (due to loss of plasma proteins). Plasma proteins are also altered in pregnancy.
- Higher doses may be needed to achieve a therapeutic effect if a drug is extensively bound. Aspirin is an example. Like many acidic drugs it binds to albumin.
- Effects may be prolonged for drugs that are highly bound because the bound drug acts as a reservoir releasing more as serum levels of free drug fall. An example is digoxin.
- Drug interaction may result from drugs competing for binding with plasma proteins. An important example is the interaction between warfarin and aspirin or warfarin and phenytoin. Usually warfarin is 97% bound to plasma proteins so there is a huge reservoir of drug that may be released to have an increased therapeutic effect.

Drug metabolism in the liver

The liver is a major site for metabolizing drugs (other sites are the gut wall, lungs, and blood plasma). The process converts the drug into a more water-soluble compound (by increasing its polarity) that can then be excreted in the body fluids, mainly urine or bile. During this process of metabolism the therapeutic effect usually diminishes. Very few drugs can be excreted without undergoing this process. Nitrous oxide, used during sedation and GA, is an example of a gas which is not metabolized.

In liver hepatocytes the smooth endoplasmic reticulum has a set of related enzymes. The main enzymes involved in metabolism of drugs belong to the cytochrome P450 group. Metabolism is divided into two phases. Most drugs undergo both phases, although some only one.

Phase 1 metabolism
- Oxidation catalysed by cytochrome P450 enzymes results in the loss of electrons from the drug.
- Alternatively phase I may involve reduction or hydrolysis of the drug.
- The resulting drug metabolite is still often chemically active.

Phase 2 metabolism
Conjugation (attachment of an ionized group to the drug, e.g. methyl, acetyl, or glutathione groups) makes the resulting metabolite more water soluble and makes it less pharmacologically active.

These metabolic processes usually occur in the hepatocyte cytoplasm. Local anaesthetics undergo a complex process of metabolism by liver microsomal enzymes.
- Phase 1 involves hydroxylation, N-dealkylation and methylation.
- Phase 2 involves conjugation with amino acids into less active and inactive metabolites. The rate of metabolism differs between agents with prilocaine being the most rapid, lidocaine and mepivacaine intermediate and bupivacaine the slowest. Prilocaine is also thought to be metabolized in the lung.

Many sedative drugs and anaesthetics undergo glucuronidation in phase 2, e.g. propofol and midazolam.

Some drug metabolites can be toxic. An example is paracetamol. The toxic metabolites are detoxified by phase 2 conjugation, joining them with glutathione. In an overdose situation there is insufficient glutathione to detoxify the paracetamol metabolites. Their accumulation can lead to hepatitis. Hence drugs are administered to increase glutathione levels so that phase 2 metabolism can continue detoxifying the paracetamol metabolites fully and reducing the risk of liver damage.

The rate of drug metabolism is affected by various factors.
- Age (generally slower in elderly)
- Gender
- Individual variation/genetic factors
- Diet and gut flora
- Pathological conditions which reduce enzyme activity, e.g. liver disease, kidney disease, reduced hepatic blood flow in heart failure or shock
- Drug interactions also have a large influence on the rate of metabolism by the microsomal enzymes. Drugs can be classed as enzyme inhibitors whereby they slow the rate of metabolism, or enzyme inducers whereby they speed up the rate of metabolism. Crucially these may result in either toxic or sub-therapeutic drug levels.

Drugs excreted into bile

Some drugs and their metabolites are extensively excreted in bile. Because they are transported across the biliary epithelium against a concentration gradient, active secretory transport is required. When plasma drug concentrations are high, secretory transport may approach an upper limit (transport maximum). Substances with similar physicochemical properties may compete for excretion.

Drugs with a molecular weight of >300 g/mol and with both polar and lipophilic groups are more likely to be excreted in bile, smaller molecules are generally excreted only in negligible amounts. Conjugation, particularly with glucuronic acid, facilitates biliary excretion.

In the enterohepatic cycle, a drug secreted in bile is reabsorbed into the circulation from the intestine. Biliary excretion eliminates substances from the body only to the extent that enterohepatic cycling is incomplete—when some of the secreted drug is not reabsorbed from the intestine. A drug excreted in bile may be reabsorbed from the GI tract or a drug conjugate may be hydrolysed by gut bacteria, liberating the original drug which can be returned to the general circulation. Cholestatic disease states, in which normal bile flow is reduced, will influence drug elimination by this route resulting in increased risk of drug toxicity.

Alcohol and the dental patient

Around 25% of adults in England have an alcohol intake at potentially or actually harmful levels increasing their risk of a wide range of medical and social problems. Potential harms include increased risk of cancers (oral, oesophageal, stomach, bowel, breast, liver), liver cirrhosis, heart disease, stroke, pancreatitis.

Alcohol recommendations

UK Chief Medical Officers recommend not regularly drinking more than 14 units of alcohol a week and that it is best to spread the units through the week. For women trying to conceive or already pregnant, it is safest to avoid alcohol totally. One unit of alcohol is defined as 10 ml of pure alcohol. So the units contained in drinks will vary with the size and strength of the drink and should be clearly indicated on product labels. For example, a glass of wine or a bottle of beer may be more than 3 units. Food in the stomach will slow absorption of alcohol and the effects will also vary with the size, gender (males process alcohol faster), general metabolic rate, health of the liver, but at a maximum the liver can metabolize 1 alcohol unit per hour. So after a night of heavy drinking, blood levels of alcohol may still be too high, the following morning, to drive legally.

Screening patients

All patients should be asked about their alcohol intake as part of routine history taking. Some screening tools have been developed, e.g. AUDIT (C): Alcohol use disorder identification test. Those found to be at risk may be given a brief advice intervention and referral to their GP or a local alcohol support service.

Clues to excess alcohol intake

In addition to direct enquiry there may be other clues, evident at a dental visit, that alcohol use is at harmful levels.
• From the history there may be social/psychological signs, e.g. anxiety, depression, relationship breakdown, work and financial problems, self-harm.
• From general observation there may also be signs of deteriorating selfcare: weight gain or weight loss, less care over appearance, signs of repeated injuries.
• From clinical examination there may be signs of: parotid enlargement (bilateral), poor oral hygiene, poor wound healing, excess bleeding, aphthae, glossitis.

'Alcohol-use disorders' is the preferred term for a range of mental health problems as recognized within the international disease classification systems (ICD-10, DSM-IV). These include:
• Hazardous drinking, which is a pattern of alcohol consumption that increases someone's risk of harm
• Harmful drinking, which is a pattern of alcohol consumption that is causing mental or physical damage

• Alcohol dependence, which is a cluster of behavioural, cognitive and physiological factors that typically include a strong desire to drink alcohol and difficulties in controlling its use. Someone who is alcohol-dependent may persist in drinking, despite harmful consequences.

Further reading

NICE. Alcohol-use disorders: prevention. Public health guideline [PH24] 2010
UK Chief Medical Officers' Low Risk Drinking Guidelines 2016. London: Crown Publishing.

Liver disease

Liver problems have been increasing and now affect around 10% of the population. Much of this is due to alcohol misuse with over 25% of the adult population drinking excessively. Obesity and diabetes play a part too. (➔ See Table 5.1)

How alcohol damages the liver

Alcohol dehydrogenase starts metabolism of alcohol in the stomach. Alcohol is then absorbed from the upper small intestine via the portal vein and transported to the liver where alcohol is converted to acetaldehyde and then excreted by conversion to carbon dioxide in the citric acid cycle. The rate of metabolism is variable, partly depending on weight, gender, and body fat. The commonly quoted rate of 1 unit per hour relates to a fit young adult male and will be slower for many. The enzymes involved in metabolizing alcohol can undergo enzyme induction and tolerance can increase.

Alcohol-related liver disease includes:
- Fatty change—reversible and the most common form
- Alcoholic hepatitis - inflammation of the liver
- Cirrhosis—irreversible changes of diffuse scarring throughout the liver and parenchymal nodules (ineffective attempts at regeneration).

These may lead onto liver failure (also called decompensation).

Causes of liver cirrhosis include:
- Alcohol-related liver disease
- Viral infection especially HBV and HCV
- Metabolic diseases iron, copper, glycogen storage disease, lipid disorders, α-1 antitrypsin deficiency
- Autoimmune disorders
- Bile duct diseases, e.g. primary biliary cirrhosis.

In 60% of the patients with alcoholic cirrhosis, bilateral parotid sialosis occurs and other glands may be affected too. Sialosis can also occur in non-alcoholic cirrhosis. Histology is of fatty infiltration, oedema, fibrosis, or acinar hypertrophy. The ducts are dilated and there is stasis of secretory granules with hypofunction and possible xerostomia.

Complications of alcohol-related liver disease

Portal hypertension and variceal bleeding

Increased resistance to portal flow secondary to scarring, narrowing, and compression of the hepatic sinusoids results in portal hypertension and varices may develop which are then prone to bleeding. Primary prophylaxis of variceal bleeding is aimed at reducing the portal pressure gradient, azygous blood flow, and variceal pressure and propranolol is the first choice drug.

Ascites

This is the pathologic accumulation of fluid in the peritoneal cavity. Spontaneous bacterial peritonitis may occur in this fluid.

Table 5.1 Some key signs of liver failure

Sign	Cause
Bleeding tendency	↓ coagulation factors, ↓ platelets, ↓ thrombopoietin, ↓ absorption of vit K
Swelling, ascites	Protein synthesis ↓ low albumin
Jaundice	Build-up of bilirubin
Itchy skin	Bile products deposited in the skin
Spider naevi on face, neck, chest and back (thin, tortuous blood vessels emanating from a central arteriole)	Unknown
Confusion	Build-up of metabolites
Nausea, fatigue, loss of appetite	Build-up of metabolites

Hepatic encephalopathy

Occurs in portal hypertension when metabolites build up and impact on brain function. Memory, personality, concentration, and reactions may be impaired.

Treatment aims to reduce the nitrogenous load and may include:

- Lactulose, a type of sugar that increases acidity in the gut to help prevent growth of some ammonia-producing bacteria
- Antibiotic (e.g. neomycin) to reduce ammonia-producing bacteria in the gut.

Hepatitis

Hepatitis is inflammation of the liver. Causes include: viruses, alcohol, drugs, and autoimmune diseases. Hepatitis may take the following forms (➲ See Table 5.2):

- Asymptomatic subclinical disease – most patients are oblivious that they have been ill
- Acute hepatitis B with clinical jaundice and full recovery
- Acute fulminant hepatitis with massive necrosis and death (<2%)
- Chronic hepatitis/carrier—lasting more than 6 months (especially hepatitis B and C) with risk of cirrhosis and hepatocellular carcinoma.

Hepatitis B

- Is an occupational hazard for health care workers
- Is 100 times more infectious than HIV
- May be acquired by blood contact, sexually transmitted, or acquired at birth from the birth canal
- Prevalence (as anti-HBs) varies widely across the world
- Prevalence of 0.01% in UK, varies across populations up to 20% in parts of Africa.

Symptoms

May be none or flu-like. (➲ See Table 5.3 and 5.4)

- Tiredness/aches and pains/fever/loss of appetite
- Nausea and vomiting and diarrhoea

Table 5.2 Types of viral hepatitis

Hepatitis A (RNA)	Faeco-oral route (2–6 weeks incubation period) usually self-limiting
Hepatitis B (DNA)	Blood-borne/sexual transmission (6 wks–6 mths incubation period)
	High risk of developing cirrhosis or liver cancer.
Hepatitis C (RNA)	Blood-borne
	(2 wks–6 months incubation period)
	~ 80% show no symptoms
	Some clear the virus spontaneously
	Risk of developing cirrhosis or liver cancer if untreated
Hepatitis D (RNA) delta agent—defective virus needs presence of HBV in order to replicate	Co-infection with HBV (at the same time or later)
	Blood-borne/sexual transmission
	There is no effective treatment
	Risk of developing cirrhosis or liver cancer if untreated
Hepatitis E (RNA)	Waterborne, mainly faecal contamination of drinking water
	(3 wks – 8 wks incubation period) usually self-limiting
Cytomegalovirus	May be a cause of hepatitis in immunocompromised patients

Table 5.3 Serological markers for Hepatitis B

Antigen	Antibody
HBsAg Hepatitis B surface antigen is the earliest indicator of acute infection. Persistence beyond 6 months of onset means chronic infection or carrier status.	**anti-HBs** This is the specific antibody to hepatitis B surface antigen. Arises from exposure to HBsAg or from vaccination. Its appearance 1–4 months after onset of symptoms indicates clinical recovery and subsequent immunity to HBV. Anti-HBs will usually not be present with HBsAg.
HBcAg Hepatitis B core antigen is derived from the protein envelope that encloses the viral DNA, and it is not detectable in the bloodstream. When HBcAg peptides are expressed on the surface of hepatocytes, they induce an immune response that is crucial for killing infected cells. The HBcAg is a marker of the infectious viral material and it is the most accurate index of viral replication.	**anti-HBc** This is the specific antibody to hepatitis B core antigen. anti-HBc indicates exposure to the hepatitis B virus and persists for many years. They do not neutralize the virus. In the absence of HBsAg and anti-HBs, it shows recent infection. Anti-HBc testing identifies all previously infected persons, including HBV carriers, but does not differentiate carriers and non-carriers. Anti-HBc does not tell you whether the patient is still infectious (HBsAg positive) or whether they have developed immunity to the virus (anti-HBs positive) since anti-HBc will be present in both conditions.
HBeAg Hepatitis B e antigen appears at weeks 3 to 6 Indicates acute active infection. Is an indicator of the patient being highly infectious. Persistence of HBeAg after 10 wks shows progression to chronic infection or carrier state.	**anti-HBe** This is the specific antibody to hepatitis B e antigen. Serology shifting from e antigen to e antibody indicates the infection is resolving. anti-HBe indicates reduced infectivity.

Table 5.4 Interpretation of the 3 standard blood tests for HBV

Clinical situation	Assay results		
	HBsAg	anti-HBs	anti-HBc
HBV infection (acute or chronic)	+	+/–	+
Past HBV infection and current immunity to HBV	–	+	+
Past HBV infection resolved/Resolving acute infection/ Low-level HBV carrier	–	–	+
Successfully vaccinated. Should give lifelong immunity if at >10 IU/mL	–	+	–

- Pale faeces, dark urine
- Jaundice (yellowing in the whites of the eyes and in skin if severe).

Treatment
- Interferon and antivirals
- Surveillance for hepatocellular carcinoma
- Liver transplantation if cirrhosis develops

Prevention
Is with inoculation of an inactivated form of HBV.
   The standard schedule is:
- Injection 1 at time zero
- Injection 2 at 1 month later
- Injection 3 at 6 months
- Blood test at 7 or 8 months (checking that >10 IU/mL anti-HBs has been achieved)
- Booster injection at 5 years
- This seems to give lifelong immunity and no further boosters are usually required.

Around 10–15% will not respond to the vaccine and they may need to repeat the process. Some may not respond to the vaccine at all.
   An accelerated schedule for vaccination is also available but gives slightly less protection.

Reye's syndrome

Reye's (Ryes) syndrome is a rare but potentially fatal condition mostly affecting children and teenagers recovering from a viral infection (flu or chickenpox). Use of aspirin in children or teenagers can also trigger the condition. Hence aspirin is not normally given to patients below the age of 16 years. The pathology is of mitochondrial dysfunction. Structural similarity has been found between aspirin metabolites and substrates for mitochondrial enzymes. Encephalopathy and fatty degeneration of liver may occur. Clinical features include diarrhoea, vomiting, seizures, and loss of consciousness requiring emergency care.

Tests for liver function

For patients who are suspected of having reduced liver function, there are a range of further investigations. (➲ See Table 5.5)

Table 5.5 Changes in blood test results in impaired liver function	
Liver function tests	
Test	Interpretation
Albumin REDUCED	Albumin, a crucial protein for maintaining osmotic pressures and for transporting many substances. Albumin production may decrease in chronic liver disease. Other causes of low serum albumin include malnutrition and protein malabsorption.
Alanine aminotransferase (ALT) increased	The aminotransferases are enzymes that are present in hepatocytes and that leak into the blood stream when liver cells are damaged. This is a sensitive marker of liver damage.
Alkaline phosphatase (ALP) increased	ALP is an enzyme found in cells of the bile duct system. Increases in ALP may indicate bile duct obstruction or other liver disease. ALP also increases in other conditions, e.g. pregnancy and bone disease, so the ALP result must be considered alongside the rest.
Serum bilirubin increased	Bilirubin is formed from breakdown of haemoglobin and is the main pigment in bile. Excess causes jaundice.
Gamma-glutamyl transferase (GGT or 'Gamma GT') increased	GGT is raised in obstructive or cholestatic liver disease, where bile is not properly transported from the liver. GGT is also a potential indicator of the patient's alcohol intake. GGT is also raised in other conditions, e.g. pancreatitis, MI, obesity, so the GGT result must be considered alongside the rest.
Aspartate aminotransferase (AST) increased	The aminotransferases are enzymes that are present in hepatocytes and that leak into the blood stream when liver cells are damaged. AST may indicate muscle damage elsewhere.
Clotting studies	
Prothrombin time (PT) prolonged	prothrombin time measures the rate of conversion of prothrombin to thrombin (II, V, VII, X and vitamin K)
International normalized ratio (INR) increased	To standardize reporting, PT results may be given as INR. It is the ratio of the patient's PT to the mean control PT.

Management of dental care in patients with impaired liver function

Patients at risk

Where impaired liver function is suspected the dentist must liaise closely with medical colleagues in caring for the patient. For patients with jaundice or a history of high alcohol intake or liver problems the patient's physician should be consulted.

An immediate concern in dental management of these patients is the increased risk of bleeding. The impact of excess alcohol is to reduce platelet numbers and impair their function. So it is recommended that a careful history of bleeding is sought.

Questions to elicit a history of bleeding

1. Do you bruise/bleed easily?
2. Does anyone in the family have problems with bleeding?
3. Ever needed medical attention due to bleeding?
4. Any nosebleeds, blood in faeces, excessive menstrual bleeding?
5. Ever had excess bleeding after tooth extraction or other surgery?

If there is a history of prolonged alcohol intake at harmful levels and a positive bleeding history then investigations may include:
1. Full blood count and coagulation screen (See Chapter 10)
2. Liver function tests

Liver-function tests are not a good predictor of how much response to a particular drug will be impaired.

In patients with impaired liver function there are 2 main concerns:

1. Bleeding tendency—coagulation factors and platelets may be reduced
- If there is doubt about liver function, liver function tests and coagulation screen should be run prior to any dental extractions or surgery.
- Intravenous vitamin K may be required if there is vitamin K malabsorption.
- Fresh frozen plasma may be needed preoperatively.
- Local haemostatic measures should be used too if excessive bleeding is a risk:

Local measures to stop bleeding
- Arrange the procedure to avoid weekends, holidays, or evenings when help may be more difficult to find
- Limit the number of teeth extracted per session
- Use a careful technique minimizing trauma
- Use LA with vasoconstrictor
- Avoid inferior alveolar nerve block injections if possible
- Gently pack the socket with absorbable dressing
- Suture the socket
- Avoid NSAIDs

Table 5.6 Drugs to avoid for patients with impaired liver function

Drug type	Specific drugs
Analgesics	NSAIDs
	Paracetamol
Antibiotics	Erythromycin
	Metronidazole
	Tetracyclines
Antifungals	Miconazole
	Fluconazole
Local anaesthetics	Any
Sedative drugs	Any

2. Drug metabolism

Drug metabolism is complicated by the liver having a reduced capacity to process drugs. In addition, plasma proteins may be reduced, interfering with binding and availability of some drugs. There may be increased sensitivity to hepatotoxic effects and to anticoagulant effects of drugs. Some drugs may also exacerbate the effects of impaired liver function such as impaired cerebral function and fluid retention. Hence, sedation or GA require specialist skills and the patient should be referred. GA in a jaundiced patient may trigger hepato-renal syndrome and renal failure. (➔ See Table 5.6)

Further reading

MacLachlan JH, Locarnini S, Cowie, BC. (2015) Estimating the global prevalence of hepatitis B. *Lancet* **386**: 1515–17.

Kidneys and chronic renal disease

The anatomy of the kidney *134*
The structure and function of the kidneys *136*
Classification of chronic renal disease *138*
Chronic kidney disease *140*
How does anaemia occur in chronic renal failure (CRF)? *142*
Bone pathology in chronic renal disease *144*
Bleeding tendency in CRF *146*
Chronic kidney disease (CKD): summary *148*

The anatomy of the kidney

Gross anatomy

The kidneys are paired organs located in the posterior part of the abdomen. They are located on either side of the midline with the centres of the kidneys lying approximately in the position of the first lumbar vertebra.

The kidneys have an outer cortex and an inner medulla.

Histological structure

➔ See Fig 6.1. The tubules consist of:
- A nephron which filters material from the plasma and selectively reabsorbs some elements
- And a series of collecting ducts which transport the urine to the pelvis of the kidney and the ureter.

Renal function

A cluster of capillary blood vessels (the glomerulus) is present in an end invagination of the tubule, called the Bowman's capsule, through which passes the plasma filtrate. The proteins and fats are prevented from passing into the tubule.

The filtration membrane is formed by:
- Fenestrations of the glomerular capillaries
- The glomerular basement membrane (formed from the endothelial cells and podocytes)
- The inner (visceral) layer of cells in the Bowman's capsule which wrap around the capillary forming podocyte processes. The slits between the processes provide an important filtration function. Damage to podocyte function causes proteinuria and renal damage.

Function of the proximal convoluted tubule

Its function is to reabsorb glucose, amino acids, and water, and sodium, phosphate, bicarbonate and chloride ions. The volume of filtrate in the tubule is reduced.

Function of the descending loop of Henle

Water is reabsorbed and the urine becomes more concentrated. Sodium permeability is low.

Function of the ascending loop of Henle

The ascending loop of Henle has two functional parts:
- The thin ascending loop allows sodium and chloride ions to passively diffuse into the tubule. Water permeability is low.
- The thick ascending loop allows active transport of sodium, potassium, and chloride ions.

This countercurrent multiplication system produces a hypertonic medulla which allows water to be reabsorbed from the collecting ducts.

Function of the distal convoluted tubule

Fine adjustment of sodium and water excretion occurs at the distal tubule and collecting ducts. Antidiuretic hormone is released by the posterior pituitary in response to osmoreceptors in the hypothalamus and acts to increase the permeability of the collecting ducts.

Aldosterone (secreted by the adrenal cortex) increases sodium reabsorption and preserves blood volume. In response to a low blood volume, renin is secreted by the juxtaglomerular apparatus, a collection of cells located near the glomerulus. Renin converts angiotensinogen to angiotensin I, which is then converted into angiotensin II. This hormone reduces glomerular filtration rate thus reducing the amount of sodium filtered by the glomerulus and also stimulates secretion of aldosterone.

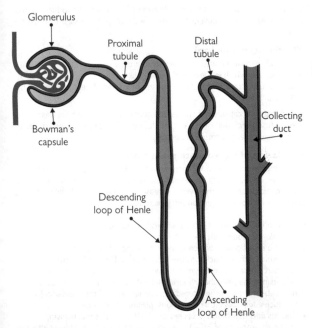

Fig. 6.1 The nephron and collecting duct system.

The structure and function of the kidneys

The kidneys remove metabolic waste products (e.g. urea), play a vital role in regulating the acidity of body fluids, and also have an endocrine function (producing erythropoietin). The kidney function is measured using the glomerular filtration rate which is the volume of plasma filtered per minute (or clearance). This can be estimated using the excretion of creatinine collected over 24 hours and using the formula:

$$\text{Clearance} = \frac{\text{Urinary concentration of creatinine} \times \text{Urinary volume} / \min}{\text{Plasma concentration of creatinine}}$$

Urinary formation results from a filtration of plasma that produces a protein free fluid that is subsequently modified during its passage through the nephron.

The filtration mechanism
The renal corpuscle consists of two structures:
- Glomerulus which is a group of capillaries
- Glomerular capsule which is composed of a layer of cells invaginated by the capillaries.

The glomerular capsule has specialized cells (podocytes) whose basal laminae are fused with that of the endothelial cells. This provides the barrier to the passage of large protein molecules.

Regulation of bicarbonate reabsorption
The kidneys can respond to changes in blood pH produced as a result of metabolic or respiratory abnormalities. With respiratory insufficiency, the pCO_2 concentration in the alveoli increases and the blood pH falls, and this stimulates active hydrogen ion (H^+) excretion.

In the tubular lumen:
- Filtered HCO_3^- cannot cross the apical membrane of the proximal convoluted tubule cells.
- Filtered bicarbonate ions combine with secreted H^+ ions to form CO_2 which diffuses back into the tubular cells. There it is converted to bicarbonate and hydrogen ions, with the former able to freely diffuse into the peritubular extracellular fluid. This mechanism causes the reabsorption of the filtered bicarbonate ions. If the tubular cells produce additional bicarbonate ions, plasma pH is raised.
- The result is that blood pH is restored. Without this mechanism, increased amounts of HCO_3^- would be lost with a net acidifying effect on the blood.

With prolonged hyperventilation at high altitude, respiratory alkalosis results, blood pH rises and is restored by the excretion of fewer hydrogen ions. The plasma concentration of bicarbonate ions falls causing a return to normal pH.

Regulation of sodium and chloride ion balance

- In the proximal convoluted tubule, sodium ions are actively transported into the peritubular fluid. The chloride ions follow passively. As the proximal tubule is freely permeable to water, the filtrate is isotonic with the blood.
- The ascending limb of the Loop of Henle is impermeable to water, but ions are actively excreted from the filtrate into the peritubular fluid. This has the effect of producing a high concentration of sodium and chloride ions in the medullary fluid.
- The fluid leaving the distal convoluted tubule is hypotonic.
- As the fluid descends through the medulla in the collecting duct, it is concentrated by water reabsorption following the osmotic gradient.
- The volume of urine formed is under the hormonal control of antidiuretic hormone (vasopressin) which controls the variable water permeability of the connecting tubules and collecting ducts. Antidiuretic hormone functions by binding aquaporin receptors on the collecting duct epithelium.

Antidiuretic hormone (vasopressin)

- Antidiuretic hormone is manufactured by the hypothalamus and stored and secreted by the posterior pituitary.
- If vascular (V1) antidiuretic hormone receptors are blocked then there is an insignificant change in arterial blood pressure. However, there may be a significant role for the hormone in providing an increased blood pressure when the function of the autonomic nervous system is impaired.

Renin–angiotensin–aldosterone system (see below)

- Aldosterone is the end product
- Aldosterone causes sodium ions and water to be reabsorbed into the peritubular extracellular fluid and increased blood pressure.

Atrial natriuretic hormone (ANP)

- Atrial natriuretic hormone is expressed by the heart in heart failure and cardiac hypertrophy. This hormone is secreted by the atria following increased wall stress as a result of a rise in the intravascular volume.
- The result of the hormone release is an increased glomerular filtration rate, diuresis, loss of sodium ions, and vasodilation.
- ANP inhibits aldosterone secretion and the sodium reabsorption action of angiotensin II.

Classification of chronic renal disease

Renal disease results from damage to nephrons which are unable to regenerate. The blood creatinine concentration can be used to estimate kidney function and glomerular filtration rate. Chronic renal disease is defined as 'severe' if the estimated glomerular filtration rate (eGFR) is 15–29 ml/minute/1.73 m^2 and 'established' (or endstage) if less than 15 ml/minute/1.73 m^2 (➔ See Table 6.1). The normal value for eGFR is 90–120 ml/min. The causative factors for chronic kidney disease (CKD) include diabetes mellitus and hypertension. Controlling the hypertension and proteinuria is important in preventing further deterioration in kidney function. The effect of kidney dysfunction is to cause a raised blood level of urea and creatinine.

Drug prescription in chronic renal failure (CRF)

In those with poor renal function, drug prescribing should be avoided where possible, especially with potentially toxic drugs that have a narrow safety margin. Prior to prescribing a drug for a patient with CRF the following important questions need to be asked:

Can the drug be excreted?

If the serum albumin is reduced, then drugs that are normally protein-bound will have an increased amount of free-drug, which may cause toxicity. This may occur with drugs such as warfarin or the benzodiazepines.

Can the drug be effective?

In chronic kidney disease, the normal metabolism of 25-hydroxycholecalciferol to the more metabolically active metabolite 1,25 dihydroxycholecalciferol (1,25-(OH)$_2$D$_3$) is reduced. The average serum concentration of the 1,25-(OH)$_2$D$_3$ is further reduced if proteinuria is present caused by the leakage of the protein into the urine.

In end-stage renal disease, the kidney is unable to excrete enough phosphate and hyperphosphataemia develops. The serum calcium concentration is low (due to the low concentration of 1,25-(OH)$_2$D$_3$) and renal osteodystrophy results.

In CRF, the hydroxylated derivatives of vitamin D (alfacalcidol and calcitriol) should be given.

Is the drug toxic?

Non-steroidal anti-inflammatory drugs should not be recommended in patients with CRF as they are nephrotoxic. Analgesic nephropathy occurs due to the analgesic abuse over many years. The kidneys undergo renal papillary necrosis and chronic interstitial nephritis. This involves atrophy of the Loop of Henle and collecting ducts with the interstitial tissue developing cellular infiltration and fibrosis.

In those with CRF, angiotensin-converting enzyme inhibitors (ACE-inhibitors), potassium-sparing diuretics and potassium supplements are toxic because the kidney with reduced function cannot reduce the raised serum potassium level which result, and this may cause heart rhythm abnormalities. Calcium channel blockers are preferred to ACE-inhibitors in treatment of renovascular hypertension.

Drugs such as penicillin and LAs are safe to use in CRF without any dose reduction. Lidocaine is metabolized by the liver and nearly two-thirds of an oral dose of amoxicillin is excreted unchanged in the urine within 8 hours of consumption. Paracetamol can be prescribed for pain relief.

Drugs where nephrotoxicity has been reported:

- Zoledronic acid (one of the bisphosphonate drugs). Where the renal function is already compromised, it needs to be closely monitored and treatment with these drugs will require a dose reduction based on the eGFR.
- Telavancin, which is used in treating hospital-acquired pneumonia, should be avoided in acute renal failure.
- Tetracyclines should be avoided as they may exacerbate renal failure.
- The antibiotics neomycin, kanamycin, and amphotericin. Patients with pre-existing renal disease develop high serum levels of these antibiotics.
- The antifungal amphotericin should only be used if there is no alternative.
- The antiviral drug aciclovir should be used at a reduced dose.

If patients with a eGFR of less than 60ml/min, are to be given non-steroidal anti-inflammatory drugs, they require the serum creatinine to be monitored as there is a potential for further renal damage.

- Non-steroidal anti-inflammatory drugs include ibuprofen, diclofenac, naproxen, and indometacin.

Table 6.1 CKD stages. (From the US National Kidney Foundation kidney disease outcomes quality initiative classification)

CKD Stage	Estimated GFR (ml/min/1.73 m²)
1 Normal	>90
2 Mildly affected function	60–89
3 Moderately reduced function	30–59
4 Severely reduced function	15–29
5 Very severely reduced function	<15

Chronic kidney disease

CKD is present when the glomerular filtration rate is less than 60 mL/min, but with patients who have only mildly reduced kidney function they may receive restorative treatment safely in general dental practice. With moderately severe kidney disease (eGFR is below 45 mL/min) the advice of the local specialist in special care dentistry should be sought.

Hepatitis C infection is the commonest cause of liver damage in patients with CKD receiving dialysis, with a resultant increased risk of mortality. Patients receiving haemodialysis are at high risk of getting a hepatitis C infection, especially where there is a high prevalence of disease in the population. Complications of hepatitis C infection include cirrhosis and hepatocellular carcinoma, but most patients on dialysis remain asymptomatic for decades. In regions affected by endemic hepatitis B infection, vaccination has reduced the spread of the infection. New anti-viral nucleos(t)ide analogs drugs (e.g. entecavir) may improve the long-term outlook of patients with chronic hepatitis B virus infection and chronic kidney disease.

Patients with chronic kidney disease often complain of
- An increased incidence of retrograde parotitis
- Chronic periodontal disease and an increased calculus formation
- An ammoniacal odour to their breath. Uraemic halitosis occurs in end-stage renal failure.

Patients with chronic kidney disease often have a reduced caries rate, probably due to the raised salivary urea.

Patients who have received a renal transplant and are taking ciclosporin have an increased incidence of gingival hyperplasia.

Diabetic nephropathy

Diabetic nephropathy is characterized by the presence of significant amounts of albumin in the urine and diabetic glomerular disease. The glomeruli undergo hypertrophy (mesangial expansion due to increased extracellular matrix production), loss of podocytes, thickening of the basement membrane, and nodular glomerulosclerosis and this is associated with renal fibrosis. The raised serum glucose concentration causes the formation of advanced glycosylated products and glomerular destruction. With activation of the renin–angiotensin system, there is narrowing of the efferent arterioles, increased hydrostatic pressure, and further albuminuria. In advanced kidney disease, there is a decrease in glomerular filtration rate and macroalbuminuria (which is excretion of albumin ≥300 mg per 24 hours) and eventually end-stage renal disease.

Renovascular hypertension

Renovascular hypertension results from reduced perfusion of the kidneys stimulating the renin–angiotensin–aldosterone system into action. The fall in renal blood flow is detected by the baroreceptors in the glomerular afferent arterioles which stimulates cells of the juxtaglomerular apparatus to produce renin. This is a collection of specialized cells that lie near the glomerulus of each nephron. Renin itself is inactive, but acts on angiotensinogen to convert it to angiotensin I, which is further metabolized by angiotensin converting enzyme (ACE) to angiotensin II, mainly in the lungs. Angiotensin II

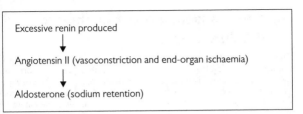

Excessive renin produced

↓

Angiotensin II (vasoconstriction and end-organ ischaemia)

↓

Aldosterone (sodium retention)

Fig. 6.2 The renin–angiotensin–aldosterone regulatory system.

is a potent vasoconstrictor and it also stimulates the adrenal cortex to produce aldosterone. The resulting effect is that the blood pressure increases
due to the increased aldosterone-induced sodium and water retention and
vasoconstriction. The vascular smooth muscle undergoes hypertrophy with
the result that there is end-organ ischaemia (➋ See Fig. 6.2).

ACE inhibitor drugs (e.g. ramipril) reduce the serum angiotensin II levels
and because less angiotensin II is produced the systemic blood vessels are
not constricted and the blood pressure falls. Angiotensin I can be converted
to angiotensin II through other mechanisms than ACE, and this can result in
poor control of hypertension in some patients. A sustained hypertension
may result in a reduction in serum renin, so measuring the output of this
hormone may not indicate renal stenosis.

Renal ischaemia causing renovascular hypertension may arise due to
atherosclerosis of the renal artery. This is becoming more common as
people live longer. Fibromuscular dysplasia affects a mainly younger female
population.

The European Medicine Agency (2014) does not recommend the combined, routine use of anti-hypertensive drugs affecting multiple points in
the renin–angiotensin–aldosterone regulatory system, especially in those
with diabetic nephropathy[1]. There are concerns that kidney function will be
impaired in those with compromised renal function. Angiotensin-receptor-
blocking drugs may increase the incidence rate of myocardial infarction (MI)
despite decreasing blood pressure[2].

References

[1] http://www.ema.europa.eu/docs/en_GB/document_library/Referrals_document/Renin-
angiotensin_system_(RAS)-acting_agents/Recommendation_provided_by_Pharmacovigilance_
Risk_Assessment_Committee/WC500165200.pdf

[2] Palmer SC, Mavridis D, Navarese E, Craig JC, Tonelli M, Salanti G, Wiebe N, Ruospo M, Wheeler
DC, Strippoli GF. (2015) Comparative efficacy and safety of blood pressure-lowering agents in
adults with diabetes and kidney disease: a network meta-analysis. *Lancet* 385:2047–56.

How does anaemia occur in chronic renal failure (CRF)?

The kidneys produce erythropoietin which is an important glycoprotein hormone in the regulation of the number of erythrocytes. The hormone has been used successfully in the treatment of anaemia in CRF. The anaemia in chronic renal disease is characterized by a reduced output of normal sized red blood cells, but the cells have a reduced survival. The nature of the toxin has not yet been identified, although the red cells oxygen carrying function is unimpaired.

Anaemia and fatigue are common complications of CRF. In published studies, it has been shown that the prevalence of anaemia increases as the mean estimated glomerular filtration rate decreases. The anaemia is further exacerbated if diabetes is also present. For the diagnosis of anaemia, a serum hemoglobin level <13.5 g/dl in men and <12.0 g/dl in women is needed[3]. Erythropoietin, a glycoprotein hormone that is produced by interstitial fibroblasts in the kidney, stimulates production of red blood cells in the bone marrow by stimulating the proliferation and differentiation of erythroid precursors. It is the deficiency of this hormone which is the main cause of anaemia in chronic kidney disease.

Hypoxia causes changes in the cell's concentration of 'hypoxia inducible factor-1' (HIF-1). The DNA transcription of erythropoietin is regulated by an adjacent hypoxia regulatory element, which is controlled by HIF-1. The proerythroblasts in the red bone marrow respond to erythropoietin by proliferating and differentiating into erythroblasts and then reticulocytes.

Synthetic forms of erythropoietin, such as darbepoetin alfa, have been used to reverse the anaemia, but trials have shown a significant risk of stroke, hypertension or other atherosclerotic complications.

Formation of RBCs

(➔ See Fig 6.3). RBCs have a lifespan of about 100–120 days. They lack a nucleus and so are unable to divide and proliferate. The earliest erythroid progenitor cell is the erythroid burst-forming unit (BFU-E), which matures to form the erythroid colony forming unit (CFU-E), which is responsive to erythropoietin. These further develop to reticulocytes and on release into the circulation become erythrocytes.

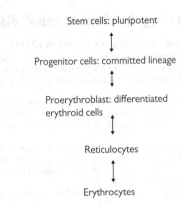

Stem cells: pluripotent

↕

Progenitor cells: committed lineage

↕

Proerythroblast: differentiated
erythroid cells

↕

Reticulocytes

↕

Erythrocytes

Fig. 6.3 Differentiation of erythrocytes from stem cells.

Clinical relevance

Bleeding in CRF
Patients with CRF are prone both to prolonged bleeding and cardiovascular complications as a result of thrombus formation.

Oral signs and symptoms of CRF undergoing dialysis.
- The mucosa can appear pale.
- Erosion of teeth due to the frequent nausea associated with haemodialysis.
- On dental radiographs there are a decreased number of bone trabeculae with thinning of the mandibular cortical border.
- Gingival enlargement due to drug therapy. Calcium-channel blockers and ciclosporin are especially likely to cause this.
- White patches and oral ulceration.

Chronic renal failure affecting children can result in enamel hypoplasia. The metabolic disturbance causes ameloblast malfunction, which results in enamel hypoplasia. This is observed as grooving or pitting of the enamel surface.

Reference

3 Macdougall IC, Eckardt KU, Locatelli F. (2007) Latest US KDOQI Anemia Guidelines update–what are the implications for Europe? *Nephrol Dial Transplant* **22**: 2738–42.

Bone pathology in chronic renal disease

Normal response of parathyroid hormone (PTH)

In health, PTH restores serum calcium to normal values. Hypocalcaemia is followed by the release of PTH from the parathyroid glands. PTH acts to restore the reduced serum calcium concentration using three main mechanisms:

1. PTH binds to the osteoblasts in bone, stimulating them to release RANKL which binds to RANK on osteoclast precursor cells causing them to differentiate into osteoclasts. Osteoclasts cause bone resorption.
2. PTH stimulates the production of 1,25-dihydroxy vitamin D, which increases the absorption of calcium ions from the gut. There is a feedback loop as 1,25-dihydroxy vitamin D suppresses PTH synthesis (independent of serum calcium).
3. PTH stimulates the reabsorption of calcium from the distal convoluted tubule.

Effect of CKD on bone

The reduced synthesis of 1,25-dihydroxy vitamin D by the kidney produces a high serum parathyroid hormone concentration. In CKD there is a high level of serum PTH driving a high bone turnover. This is seen as a high rate of bone formation and resorption. Alternatively, a mineralization defect and osteomalacia or even a mixed picture (producing a mixed renal osteodystrophy) can be present. From knowledge of the role of PTH in normal calcium metabolism, it could be conjectured that the high serum PTH concentration was triggered by hypocalcaemia. However, in CKD low serum calcium is not common or a necessary prerequisite for secondary hyperparathyroidism. It is the inability of the kidneys to excrete sufficient phosphate which leads to elevated serum levels and secondary hyperparathyroidism. In CRF, dietary phosphate restriction and drug therapy are used to reduce the serum PTH level.

Secondary hyperparathyroidism in CKD may lead to an increased risk of bone fractures, vascular calcification, and cardiovascular disease. Vascular calcification is associated with increased stiffness of the arterial wall, hypertension, and an increased mortality.

Giant cell lesions of the jaw can complicate CKD.

Chronic kidney disease patients treated by dialysis can have a mixed picture of low and high bone turnover disease (renal osteodystrophy). However, the term 'CKD-mineral and bone disorder (CKD-MBD)' is now preferred to describe the broader clinical syndrome and 'renal osteodystrophy' is used to describe the bone morphology.

Table 6.2 The different effects of bone formation and resorption on secondary hyperparathyroidism and osteomalacia

	Bone formation	Bone resorption
Secondary hyperparathyroidism	Increased	Increased
Osteomalacia	Decreased	Decreased

Bone changes following kidney transplantation

In those who have received a successful kidney transplant, bone metabolism may continue to be affected by:

- High doses of corticosteroid that are used for immunosuppression
- Continued hyperparathyroidism.

Adverse bone changes can occur despite a return to normal kidney function. A minority of kidney transplant patients can develop persistent hyperparathyroidism, hypercalcaemia and osteoporotic bone loss.

High dose corticosteroid therapy

Dentists should be aware of the potential risk of secondary osteoporosis in patients receiving high doses of glucocorticoid. Affected patients have an increased risk of bone fractures.

Glucocorticoids have:

- The majority of their effect by inducing a reduction in osteoblast number and function (causing reduced bone formation).
- There is also a more minor effect due to the stimulated expression of RANK-ligand (which increases osteoclastic bone resorption).

Patients with osteoporosis may be diagnosed from changes observed in the dental radiographs. These may be:

- Reduced thickness of the inferior cortical border of the mandible
- Increased porosity of the inferior cortical border
- Increased radiolucency of the mandibular trabecular bone.

Bleeding tendency in CRF

The treatment of patients with end stage renal disease undergoing regular dialysis can be influenced by severe bleeding during oral surgery. The detailed mechanisms are not fully understood but it is thought to be due to both a platelet dysfunction, aggregation, and an abnormality of the vessel walls.

Recommendation 1: Oral surgery treatment

1. Patients with CRF should undergo oral surgery on the day after dialysis because the adverse effect of the uraemia on blood clotting will be corrected.
2. Excessive bleeding is more common in patients with elevated serum creatinine (>1.5 mg/dL). Normal values of serum creatinine are 0.6–1.2 mg/dL in adult males and 0.5 to 1.1 mg/dL in females. Surgery should avoid excessive tissue damage with careful suturing and the application of post-operative pressure packs.

Excessive bleeding may be tested for using skin bleeding time. It is a useful and simple test in predicting the risk of bleeding prior to surgery.

Effect of uraemic toxins

- Uraemic toxins play a causative role in the increased bleeding time
- Bleeding time is improved following dialysis treatments
- The average platelet lifespan is reduced in patients with severe uraemia.

Abnormal bleeding

This is due to a defect in the formation of the platelet plug as the platelets have defective adhesion with the endothelium of the vessel wall.

Various theories exist to explain the bleeding tendency

- A dysfunctional interaction between platelet binding and von Willebrand factor
- Inhibition of platelets by nitric oxide produced by the injured vessel wall.
- Anaemia. It is postulated that in anaemia (a common complication of CRF) the platelets circulate away from the periphery of the vessel wall. This interferes with the formation of the platelet plug. The bleeding time is improved when the haematocrit is raised to 30%. This value is still below the normal range (about 42–54% for males and 38–46% for women). Recombinant erythropoietin is effective in reducing the bleeding time. However, providing a normal haematocrit in these patients is associated with an increased incidence of MI.

In determining whether a patient with CRF has an altered haemostatic state, it is important to note that the plasma coagulation factors and those governing fibrinolysis are unaltered.

Recommendation 2: Providing routine dental treatment

1. This is essential in maintaining the dental and oral health of the patient with chronic renal disease.
2. Oral hygiene instruction is indispensable, especially in those taking either ciclosporin and/or calcium-blocking agents where the patients have an increased risk of gingival hypertrophy.
3. Periodontal probing, endodontics, supragingival scaling and polishing, prosthodontics, and general restorative procedures can be undertaken without the risk of significant bleeding.

Chronic kidney disease (CKD): summary

Commonest cause of CKD is diabetes mellitus. Patients with chronic renal disease may have:

- Bleeding tendency
- Hypertension (high blood pressure) may be a factor in causing CKD, but is also a feature of the disease
- Increased risk of cardiovascular disease caused by atherosclerosis
- Anaemia due to decreased erythropoietin synthesis
- The reduced synthesis of 1,25-dihydroxy vitamin D by the kidney causes a reduced amount of calcium absorption from the kidney. Secondary hyperparathyroidism and other disturbances in mineral and bone metabolism can result.
- Metabolic acidosis.

Recommendation 3: Clinical relevance summary

1. Local anaesthetic agents and intravenous induction agents (e.g. propofol) are generally considered safe
2. Metronidazole can be given at normal dose to patients with CKD.
3. Paracetamol can be given at the normal standard dose to relieve pain. The reported adverse effects of long-term paracetamol useage are disputed and further research is needed.

Further reading

Waddington F, Naunton M, Thomas J. (2014) Paracetamol and analgesic nephropathy: Are you kidneying me? *Int Med Case Rep J.* 8:1–5.

Diabetes

The anatomy of the pancreas *150*
How is the glucose concentration in the blood monitored? *152*
Insulin resistance *156*
Epidemiology of diabetes *158*
Medical complications of diabetes *160*
Dental complications of diabetes *162*
Poorly controlled diabetic patients and infection *164*
Diabetes and severe infection *166*
Summary *168*

The anatomy of the pancreas

The pancreas has two main functions
- Digestive function secreting enzymes into the duodenum
- Role in secreting insulin, glucagon, somatostatin, and pancreatic polypeptide.

Gross anatomy

The pancreas lies in the upper part of the abdomen. The pancreas is usually described as having head (nearest the duodenum), body, and tail regions. The tail of the pancreas extends laterally towards the spleen and lies dorsal to the stomach.

The blood supply of the pancreas is provided by pancreatic branches of the splenic artery. The detailed arterial blood supply to the pancreas is very complex with many anatomical variations[1].

Venous blood drains into the portal and splenic veins.

Function of the pancreas

Exocrine function

In its exocrine function, digestive enzymes are secreted by acinar cells into the acinar tubules. The enzymes then flow into intralobular ducts, which join with interlobular ducts and finally the main pancreatic duct. Leakage of the digestive enzymes into the surrounding interstitial space is prevented by tight intercellular junctions between the acinar cells and a thick protective collagen wall surrounds the main and interlobular ducts.

The digestive enzymes are:
- Amylase (hydrolyses starch, converting it into disaccharides and trisaccharides)
- Lipase (hydrolyses fat)
- Proteases (trypsin and chymotrypsin which hydrolyse proteins and are activated by enterokinase, an enzyme produced in the mucosal cells of the duodenum and proximal jejunum
- Other enzymes.

Endocrine function

In the pancreas, the cells in the islets of Langerhans produce the following hormones that are then secreted into the blood:
- β-cells produce insulin
- α-cells produce glucagon (which increases blood glucose)
- δ-cells produce somatostatin (which inhibits insulin release)
- ε-cells produce the hormone ghrelin (increases hunger by acting on the hypothalamic cells). Ghrelin has an antagonistic effect to leptin (which stimulates a feeling of satiety in the hypothalamus).

Pancreatic polypeptide is produced in the islets of Langerhans. Its function may be to regulate food intake as the plasma concentration is elevated in anorexia nervosa.

With hypoglycaemia, glucagon is normally secreted and stimulates the breakdown of glycogen in the liver. Gluconeogenesis, the formation of glucose from non-carbohydrate precursors such as amino acids, is also stimulated. Insulin and somatostatin inhibit glucagon secretion. Following the deficient insulin secretion in diabetes, there is an increased alpha-cell activity and excess glucagon is secreted. The glucagon therefore contributes to the hyperglycaemia that characterizes diabetes. The increased glucagon secretion in diabetes type II may be responsible for a substantial rise in the serum glucose concentration following glucose intake[2].

α-cell tumours of the pancreas produce diabetes mellitus which is in agreement with the hypothesis that excess glucagon secretion may play a minor role in the onset of diabetes. Early insulin resistance in the skeletal muscle, adipocytes, and liver is traditionally thought of as the primary factor in causing hyperglycaemia which with declining insulin secretion eventually develops into type II diabetes.

Clinical implications: pancreatic cancer

Pancreatic cancer has a poor survival rate at 5 years post diagnosis. Radiotherapy and chemotherapy are not generally effective. Surgery (such as Whipple's procedure for cancer involving the head of the pancreas) has a poor survival rate. Carcinoma affecting the head of the pancreas can cause jaundice due to obstruction of the bile duct, but pain is more likely to be a presenting symptom when localized to the body or tail of the pancreas.

Tumours of the islets of Langerhans that secrete insulin are termed insulinomas. These patients suffer from fasting hypoglycaemia that is relieved by glucose.

References

1 Okahara M, Mori H, Kiyosue H, Yamada Y, Sagara Y, Matsumoto S. Arterial supply to the pancreas; variations and cross-sectional anatomy. (2010) *Abdom Imaging*. **35**:134–42.
2 Shah P, Vella A, Basu A, Basu R, Schwenk WF, Rizza RA. (2000) Lack of suppression of glucagon contributes to postprandial hyperglycemia in subjects with type 2 diabetes mellitus. *J Clin Endocrinol Metab*. **85**:4053–9.

How is the glucose concentration in the blood monitored?

In Type I diabetes there is auto-immune damage to the pancreatic β-cells of the islets of Langerhans which produce insulin in response to a raised glucose concentration in the blood. Following a glucose drink, the glucose is transported into the β-cell where the glycolysis increases the concentration of adenosine triphosphate. This causes the blockage of the ATP-dependent K^+ channels, membrane depolarization, and activation of voltage-gated Ca^{2+} channels. The cell concentration of Ca^{2+} increases which causes the insulin-containing secretory granules to undergo exocytosis. The rate of conversion of glucose to pyruvate by glucokinase in the β-cell is the crucial, rate-limiting step that controls the response to the rising glucose concentration in the blood.

Glycation end products

Advanced glycation end products (AGEs) are formed as a result of hyperglycaemia and are thought to have many harmful effects, e.g. cardiovascular disease, retinopathy, and nephropathy. Glycation of the lens proteins in diabetic patients causes cataract formation.

Glycated haemoglobin (HbA1c) is formed by non-enzymatic glycation of haemoglobin and is therefore a measure of the patient's glycaemic control over the previous 8–12 weeks. The normal range of HbA_{1c} is 20–40 mmol/mol (4–5.8% Diabetes Control and Complications Trial or DCCT units), with values greater than 48 mmoles/mol (6.5% DCCT) diagnosing diabetes[1]. The test does not require the patient to fast. The American Diabetes Association recommends that the HbA1c be maintained below 53 mmol/mol (7.0% DCCT) for most patients as being a realistic goal but which will reduce the incidence rate of macrovascular complications[2]. (➔ See Table 7.1)

Table 7.1. Significance of glycated haemoglobin (HbA1c) level in determining a diabetic diagnosis

HbA1c level (mmoles/mol)	HbA1c level (mmol/l)	Diagnosis
38.8–46.6	6.5–7.6	At risk of diabetes
42.1–47.5	7.0–7.7	At high risk of diabetes
48	>7.7	Diagnosed diabetic

Type I and type II Diabetes

Diabetes is characterized by a raised blood glucose level caused by either a reduced secretion of insulin or a failure in the metabolic action of insulin[3]. (➲ See Table 7.2)

The symptoms of diabetes include excessive thirst (polydipsia), an excessive production of urine (polyuria), tiredness, and unexplained weight loss.

Glucose intolerance is a general term to describe those conditions giving rise to raised blood glucose levels. Insulin is unable to control the production of glucose by the liver and increase the glucose uptake by peripheral tissues such as skeletal muscle. However, with post-prandial hyperglycaemia the utilization of glucose by skeletal muscle tissue in diabetes is normal and is caused by the increased glucose concentration. Because of reduced insulin secretion and increased hepatic insulin resistance, the postprandial hyperglycaemia is triggered by the inability to limit endogenous hepatic glucose production.

The severity of presentation of type I and type II diabetes can overlap, so practical distinction between the two types can be difficult. Type I diabetes is caused by the auto-immune destruction of the β-cells in the pancreas and usually develops in children but can occur at any age. Peak age of onset is 12 years. The aetiology of the disease has a genetic component, with an increased risk if siblings or parents are affected.

Type I diabetes is insulin dependent with β-cell antibodies, whereas Type II diabetes is characterized by insulin resistance and patient obesity. The aim of treatment should be to maintain blood glucose in the range 4.5–7 mmol/l, with the post-prandial glucose limited to increases to 8–10 mmol/l.

Table 7.2. Diabetes is associated with a raised plasma glucose

Normal individual: venous plasma glucose (mmoles/l)	Diabetic individual: venous plasma glucose (mmoles/l)
After fasting: <6.1	After fasting ≥7.0
*2 h after a glucose drink: <7.8	*2 h after a glucose drink >11.1
No symptoms of hyperglycaemia	Symptoms of hyperglycaemia and plasma glucose ≥11.1 mmol/l in measurement taken without regard to time since the last meal

*Following the administration of an oral glucose tolerance test. This involves giving 75 g of anhydrous glucose dissolved in water.

Glucose tolerance test

An oral glucose tolerance test could be used when the blood test results are not definitive, e.g. when the fasting level of blood glucose is between 5.5 and 6.9 mmol/l or a random test shows that the blood glucose is unusually raised at between 5.5 and 11.0 mmol/l. The patient should have fasted for 10–12 hours, although water is permitted. The test involves taking venous blood at baseline and after 2 hours.

After fasting for 10 hours prior to the test, 75 g anhydrous glucose is administered. The normal fasting blood glucose is about 3.5–5.5 mmol/l and at 2 hours the glucose level should be <7.8 mmol/l as a result of the increased insulin secretion. In the diabetic patient it is higher (>7 mmol/l) and after 2 hours, it is raised to >11.1 mmol/l. (➔ See Fig 7.1)

The glucose tolerance test will, by itself, not allow the physician to diagnose whether the patient has a type I or II diabetic condition. Type I diabetes is characterized by an insufficient secretory response of insulin following a rising glucose blood level. In type II diabetes, there is both a reduced secretion of insulin and an impaired response of the cells to insulin (called insulin resistance).

Time (mins)	Normal glucose (mmol/l)	Diabetic glucose (mmol/l)
0	5	8
30	5.5	9
60	7	10
120	5	13

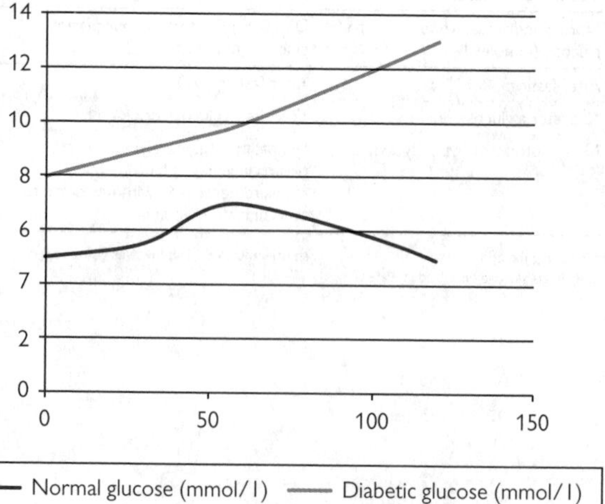

Fig. 7.1 Diagrammatic representation of glucose tolerance test.

Acute symptoms of diabetes

Hypoglycaemia

To prevent hypoglycaemia, the patient should be encouraged to eat meals at regular intervals. These should involve a low fat and sugar content, but include adequate quantities of fruit and vegetables.

Hypoglycaemia occurs when the blood glucose falls below 3.9 mmol/l. Symptoms can be thought of as the result of the body's attempt to raise the blood glucose through release of catecholamines.

- The patient may appear sweaty and pale
- Raised heart rate and a rapid pulse
- Tremor
- Patient may behave aggressively or in acute hypoglycaemia fail to respond to commands.

At blood glucose levels of 1.5mmol/L, hypoglycaemia is severe and the patient is unconscious.

Treatment involves giving the conscious patient 10–20 g of glucose orally or if the patient is unconscious injecting 1 mg of glucagon intramuscularly.

Hyperglycaemia

Symptoms of diabetic ketoacidosis (hyperglycaemia) include:

- Ketotic smell to the breath
- Acidosis.

The autonomic symptoms of hyperglycaemia are the opposite of that of hypoglycaemia with dry skin and a weak pulse. The ketoacidosis is caused by the lipolysis which releases fatty acids into the circulation. This stimulates Kussmaul breathing, which reduces the plasma bicarbonate. There is glucosuria, an osmotic diuresis, which reduces the high serum glucose with consequent dehydration. The condition progresses with hypotension and impaired glomerular filtration. Complications may rarely include cerebral oedema.

References

[3] WHO. Use of Glycated Haemoglobin (HbA1c) in the Diagnosis of Diabetes Mellitus; World Health Organization, 2011.

[4] American Diabetes Association (2009) Executive Summary: Standards of medical care in diabetes—2009. *Diabetes Care* **32**: S6–S12.

[5] American Diabetes Association. (2008) Diagnosis and classification of diabetes mellitus. *Diabetes Care* **31**: S55–S60.

Insulin resistance

Type II diabetes is caused by a reduction in beta cell function and insulin sensitivity. An increased resistance to glucose uptake by the tissues is present in the majority of type II diabetic patients. Chronic hyperglycaemia has a toxic effect and reduces the number of β-cells, which tends to cause a further reduction in insulin secretion. Long-term hyperglycaemia causes chronic oxidative stress in the β-cells resulting in apoptosis[6].

The chronic exposure of the β-cells to high blood concentrations of free fatty acids also reduces the insulin secretion through the accumulation in the cells of the toxic products of lipid metabolism. The reduced sensitivity of cells to insulin increases the demand on the β-cells to produce more insulin which leads the cells to become exhausted and eventually undergo apoptosis.

Insulin resistance is the reduced ability of insulin to increase glucose transport into adipocytes, skeletal muscle, and liver cells, and stimulate intracellular glucose metabolism. Obesity causes an increased resistance to insulin with a corresponding increase in insulin secretion, but this can be reversed by weight loss and exercise. When resistance to insulin is increased, glucose tolerance remains normal only if there is also a compensatory increase in insulin secretion. With an inadequate insulin response, Type II diabetes results. The matched relationship between insulin resistance and secretion is unlikely to be controlled by the blood glucose level, but insulin resistance may cause increased activity in the vagus nerve which stimulates an insulin response[7].

Which tissue is responsible for glucose resistance?

Skeletal muscle and the liver are the main tissues that normally act under the influence of insulin to reduce the blood glucose following a meal. In adipose tissue, insulin increases glucose uptake and inhibits lipolysis. In insulin resistance, glycogen synthesis is impaired by inhibition of the glycogen synthase enzyme. Insulin resistance develops in skeletal muscle and liver, but also occurs in the heart and adipose tissue[8].

Good glycaemic control

The aim is to prevent the 'at risk' patient becoming a type II diabetic with its associated risk of:
- Blindness
- Kidney damage
- Neuropathy
- Foot ulceration
- Blood vessel disease especially affecting the coronary arteries.

Good glycaemic control reduces the risk of diabetic microvascular complications (e.g. diabetic retinopathy).

Dentists in primary care should be involved in offering assessments for patients at risk of developing type II diabetes, using questionnaires such as the 'Diabetes Risk Score assessment tool,' (see https://www.diabetes.org.uk/Professionals/Diabetes-Risk-Score-assessment-tool/). This validated

questionnaire uses risk factors of age, gender, waist circumference, BMI, ethnicity, blood pressure, and family history to develop a numerical score.
- When someone who is at low risk is identified then advice about diet and getting exercise may still be appropriate.
- Patients with high and moderate risk scores should be referred to their general medical practitioner for further management. This may involve further tests such as fasting plasma glucose, HbA$_{1c}$ level, or an oral glucose tolerance test.

For those patients with a high score on the questionnaire, but with fasting plasma glucose between 5.5 and 6.9 mol/l (or HBA$_{1c}$ of 42–47 mmol/l) they should be referred to an intense lifestyle change programme delivering empathetic messages about exercise, weight management, and dietary advice.

Factors predictive of complications

The level of HbA1c indicates the average blood glucose and therefore assesses the patient's metabolic control over the previous month. The HbA1c level should be maintained at less than 7.7–9.3 mmol/l to prevent complications, but those at risk of hypoglycaemia may be advised to maintain a value towards the higher end of this range.

References

6 Robertson RP, Harman J, Tran PO, Tanaka Y, Takahashi H. (2003) Glucose toxicity in beta-cells: type 2 diabetes, good radicals gone bad, and the glutathione connection. *Diabetes* **52**:581–7.

7 Ahrén B, Pacini G. (2004) Importance of quantifying insulin secretion in relation to insulin sensitivity to accurately assess beta cell function in clinical studies. *Eur J Endocrinol* **150**:97–104.

8 Saltiel AR, Kahn CR. (2001) Insulin signaling and regulation of glucose and lipid metabolism. *Nature* **414**:799–806.

Epidemiology of diabetes

The scale of the problem

At present, there are nearly 4 million people in the UK with either diagnosed or undiagnosed diabetes. This is about 6% of the population with more women affected by obesity than men. The rising incidence of diabetes type II and its complications are due to an epidemic of obesity in the general population. In Western Europe, the proportion of the population with obesity increases with age until about 50–60 years of age. At present, slightly over 20% of the UK population is obese. Obesity is associated with a significantly increased risk of premature death.

The increasing incidence of diabetes type II is related to a parallel increase in obesity which is associated with the consumption of foods high in calorific value and a sedentary lifestyle.

How is obesity defined?

Obesity is defined using BMI. This is calculated by dividing an individual's weight (in kg) by the square of their height (in m^2). (➔ See Table 7.3)

As well as an increased risk of diabetes type II, obesity is associated with an increased risk of cardiovascular disease, cancers (such as prostate, breast, and ovarian cancers), and hypertension.

Central obesity

BMI is a convenient measure of obesity, but it is unable to describe the distribution of adipose tissue or its type. The accumulation of visceral adipose tissue in the abdominal area rather than its overall amount is a better predictor of glucose intolerance and type II diabetes mellitus.

Several mechanisms have been proposed to explain the link between central obesity and diabetes mellitus. The adipocytes in the visceral fat are thought to be dysfunctional and release free fatty acids and inflammatory cytokines into the portal circulation. This causes increased hepatic insulin resistance and increased hepatic glucose production (gluconeogenesis). A reduced hepatic clearance of insulin is also thought to contribute to hyperinsulinaemia which, in its turn, also contributes to systemic insulin resistance.

Table 7.3 BMI	
BMI (kg/m2)	Diagnosis
30 and over	Obese
25–30	Overweight
18.5–25	Normal weight
Under 18.5	Underweight

Dental health in type 1 diabetic children

In the literature, there is little demonstrable difference in the caries experience of children with type 1 diabetes and healthy controls. It would appear that these children develop dietary strategies early in life. These children tend to have more frequent meals but also substitute a diet rich in sugar (a cariogenic diet) for a more caries preventative diet. Caries will be reduced in a controlled diet containing a reduced amount of sugar.

Hyposalivation may be seen in diabetic patients and this may contribute to the caries incidence.

Medical complications of diabetes

(● See Table 7.4) The devastating vascular complications of diabetes are the result of the chronic hyperlipidaemia and hyperglycaemia. These cause an increase in the oxidative stress, i.e. reactive oxygen species (ROS) such as superoxide anions (O_2^-) in the endothelium, which trigger a series of biochemical events culminating in inflammation and cell death (apoptosis). Increased levels of serum free fatty acid can cause endothelial damage by increasing apoptosis. The result is that the endothelium becomes prone to develop atherosclerosis.

Obesity is known to be a risk factor for type II diabetes and vascular disease. Adipocytes release pro-inflammatory cytokines which contribute to the vascular dysfunction.

Macrovascular complications

These are complications affecting the large arteries of the heart, brain, and legs. There is therefore an increased risk of MI, stroke, and peripheral vascular disease.

Prevention of stroke involves:
• Controlling hypertension when present
• Giving antiplatelet drugs
• Smoking cessation.

It is controversial whether there is any reduced incidence of cardiovascular disease from intensive glycaemic control in patients with established type 2 diabetes mellitus[9].

Microvascular complications

The major complications are retinopathy and nephropathy.

Retinopathy

The incidence of retinopathy increases with hypertension and increasing duration and levels of hyperglycaemia. It is therefore more prevalent amongst the older patients with type I diabetes. Values above 6.5 mmol/l for fasting plasma glucose and 6.5% for HbA1c are predictive of diabetes-specific retinopathy[10].

Table 7.4 Insulin effects

Role of insulin in health	Observed effect in diabetes
Causes an uptake of glucose into the tissues	Hyperglycaemia
Promotes protein synthesis	Weight loss and reduced protein synthesis
Inhibits lipolysis and increases uptake of free fatty acids into the adipose tissues	Hyperlipidaemia (high serum free fatty acids)

Diabetic retinopathy can progress to blindness and is characterized by haemorrhage, microaneurysms, and occlusion of the retinal capillaries. It may diagnosed as:

- Non-proliferative diabetic retinopathy. This is caused by abnormalities in the leukocytes and pericytes surrounding the capillaries which result in microaneurysms and haemorrhages.
- Proliferative diabetic retinopathy: caused by the formation of new blood vessels. There is a risk of haemorrhage of these new blood vessels and blindness.
- Cataract. This is a clouding of the lens with visual impairment.
- Glaucoma. The raised intra-ocular pressure can lead to blindness.

Diabetic nephropathy

Those with early onset diabetes have an increased risk of death from diabetic nephropathy and cardiovascular disease. The accumulated changes in diabetic nephropathy have a complex aetiology. Diabetic nephropathy arises from dilation of the arteriole leading into the glomerulus, which raises the filtration pressure. Increased permeability to protein results from progressive damage to the glomerular capillaries and thickening of the glomerular basement membrane. The protein filtrate may provoke tubular interstitial damage and tubular atrophy[11].

Advanced glycation product formation on matrix proteins may exacerbate diabetic glomerulosclerosis and vascular damage. These changes, together with production of pro-inflammatory cytokines and macrophage infiltration, result in albuminuria[12].

References

9 Green JB. (2014) Understanding the type 2 diabetes mellitus and cardiovascular disease risk paradox. *Postgrad Med.* **126**:190–204.

10 Colagiuri S1, Lee CM, Wong TY, Balkau B, Shaw JE, Borch-Johnsen K, DETECT-2 Collaboration Writing Group. (2011) Glycemic thresholds for diabetes-specific retinopathy: implications for diagnostic criteria for diabetes. *Diabetes Care* **34**:145–50.

11 Abbate M, Zoja C, Remuzzi G (2006) How does proteinuria cause progressive renal damage? *J Am Soc Nephrol* **17**:2974–84.

12 Sun YM, Su Y, Li J, Wang LF. (2013) Recent advances in understanding the biochemical and molecular mechanism of diabetic nephropathy. *Biochem Biophys Res Commun.*; **433**:359–.

Dental complications of diabetes

Periodontal disease and diabetes

There is a close relationship between diabetes and periodontal disease with a high prevalence of periodontal disease amongst patients with diabetes. A similar increased prevalence of peri-implantitis has been found in diabetic patients. Poor glycaemic control is associated with chronic periodontitis with progressive alveolar bone loss[14].

One explanation may be that obesity is a risk factor for type II diabetes and may also be associated with the release of pro-inflammatory factors by adipocytes which act to modify the host response in periodontal disease[15].

Alternatively, diabetes may be associated with an altered inflammatory response or impaired collagen metabolism which is unable to respond as previously to a bacterial challenge[16].

In this situation, the level of bacterial plaque may not correspond with the severity of the periodontal disease.

The inflammation associated with chronic periodontitis may exacerbate insulin resistance. The mechanism may be through circulating cytokine reducing the secretion of insulin from the beta cells with a resulting increased insulin tolerance. A Cochrane review suggests that there may be a small beneficial effect on the control of the blood glucose from treating periodontal disease in those with Type 2 diabetes[17].

Particular emphasis should therefore be placed in maintaining periodontal health as one way of improving glycaemic control. Currently, research is ongoing into whether advanced glycation products and periodontal infection are synergistic in causing the severe periodontal destruction and atherosclerotic complications of diabetes.

Diabetes and endodontic disease

There is some evidence of a greater prevalence of periapical lesions of teeth and severity of endodontic infections in diabetic patients than non-diabetic patients.

Poorly controlled diabetic patients and dry mouth

Hyperglycaemia causes a loss of glucose in the urine which is accompanied by an increase in the volume and frequency of micturition. The increase in plasma osmolality stimulates the patient to drink water frequently. If the patient drinks fruit juice instead of water, then this will further impair their glycaemic control and increase the caries risk.

The dry mouth may cause an increased risk of dental caries, due to the lack of salivary remineralization of early carious lesions, and candidiasis. The incidence of carious lesions can be reduced by using toothpaste with 5,000ppm fluoride, professional three-monthly application of fluoride varnish, and diet advice. Sugar-free chewing gum may be helpful in some patients. Oral candidiasis should be treated with anti-fungal agents.

Amongst patients with diabetes, there is an increased prevalence of burning and tingling sensations in their mouth, diagnosed as 'burning mouth syndrome or oral dysaesthesia'. The aetiology is complex and poorly understood, but may be considered a neuropathy. Moore et al (2007) found an increased incidence of burning mouth syndrome amongst diabetic women with peripheral neuropathy[18].

Both conditions have similarities in that pain is often the presenting symptom with a complete absence of objective clinical signs. Scardina et al (2009) observed an increased mucosal capillary diameter in diabetic patients, although this may be the result of micro-inflammation rather than the cause of burning mouth syndrome. Measurements were performed using videocapillaroscopic examination in a small sample of patients with burning mouth syndrome (n=14)[19].

Oral candidiasis

Patients with **uncontrolled** diabetes are prone to candidal infection, especially if the patient is a denture wearer. The number of candidal organisms is increased in those with poor denture hygiene or who wear dentures at night. Studies which have tested whether there is a correlation between diabetes and oral candidiasis have produced conflicting results. This is due to the heterogeneous methods of sampling the *Candida* and measuring the severity of diabetes. Even if an increased number of candidal organisms are shown to be present in well-controlled diabetes, there is little evidence that this translates into an increased risk of candidal infection. Data from diabetic animal experiments and patients with poor glycaemic control indicate that they are predisposed to candidal infection.

Because patients with diabetes may be more prone to candidal infections, they may be more likely to present with the following candida-related conditions: angular cheilitis, median rhomboid glossitis, and chronic atrophic candidiasis. The reason for the increased risk of oral candidiasis may be due to the dry mouth and reduced candidal clearance, or reduced leukocytic phagocytic activity.

References

14 Taylor GW, Burt BA, Becker MP, Genco RJ, Shlossman M. (1998) Glycemic control and alveolar bone loss progression in type 2 diabetes. *Ann Periodontol.* 3:30–9.

15 Levine RS. (2013) Obesity, diabetes and periodontitis—a triangular relationship? *Br Dent J* 215:35–9.

16 Leite RS, Marlow NM, Fernandes JK. Oral health and type 2 diabetes. (2013) *Am J Med Sci* 345:271–3.

17 Simpson TC, Needleman I, Wild SH, Moles DR, Mills EJ. Treatment of periodontal disease for glycaemic control in people with diabetes. Cochrane Database of Systematic Reviews 2010, Issue 5. Art. No.: CD004714.

18 Moore PA, Guggenheimer J, Orchard T. (2007) Burning mouth syndrome and peripheral neuropathy in patients with type 1 diabetes mellitus. *Diabetes Complications* 21:397–402.

19 Scardina GA, Pisano T, Carini F, Valenza V, Messina P. (2008) Burning mouth syndrome: an evaluation of in vivo microcirculation. *JADA* 139:940–946.

Poorly controlled diabetic patients and infection

Streptozotocin is a diabetogenic drug which has been used to provide an animal model of severe uncontrolled diabetes. This drug selectively destroys the β-cells of the islets of Langerhans. The resulting hyperglycaemia has been used to study calvarial wound healing, where there is production of a plentiful, primitive woven bone and persistence of necrotic bone on the periphery of the wound. Remodelling of bone following trauma is impaired in this animal model of bone healing and this may be due to an abnormal micro-vascular response. This may explain the poor bone contact resulting from implant placement in uncontrolled diabetes[20].

Animal models

Animal models of type II diabetes have produced similar results showing an inhibition of bone contact around implants[21].

However, when the healing of tooth extraction wounds was studied in the diabetic rat model, no evidence of disordered angiogenesis was observed. In these studies, bacterial plaque on the exposed bone surface, defective epithelial proliferation, poor collagen formation, and a dense infiltrate of polymorphonuclear leucocytes all contributed to a delayed bone formation in the diabetic extraction socket[22].

The collagen fibres are especially important in the early stages of normal extraction socket healing as they form a network onto which the trabeculae of woven bone are formed. The defective development of the collagen fibres in the socket may therefore delay the establishment of the woven bone. Reduced amounts of collagen and bone matrix proteins have been described in diabetic murine models of long bone healing. The differentiation of osteoprogenitor cells to osteoblasts is attenuated in diabetes and reversed by insulin treatment[23].

Clinical studies

In diabetic patients, infection causes an increased requirement for insulin secretion. This is because the stress response is to release adrenaline and cortisol which tend to produce hyperglycaemia. 'Well-controlled' diabetes is not a contraindication to surgery such as implant placement, but this term is not well defined in the literature. In addition, many of the published clinical trials involved small numbers of diabetic patients and were of a retrospective design, with its many attendant biases. A systematic review of implant failure rate in diabetic patients showed that they did not have a higher implant failure rate than non-diabetic patients (risk ratio = 1.07)[24]; Also 'fairly well controlled' diabetic patients (i.e. with a HbA1c = 7% to 9%) did not have a higher implant failure rate[25].

This may seem surprising given the widespread deleterious effects of uncontrolled diabetes observed in the animal experiments, but the differences observed between animal experiments and clinical trials probably relate to the level of glycaemic control. The clinical study by Oates et al (2009) supported this conclusion when it reported that implant stability required a longer healing period in those type 2 diabetic patients with a HbA1c >8.1%.

General conclusions

Wound healing is delayed in diabetic patients.

The reasons for this include a failure of the early inflammatory stage responses to eliminate the infection due to:

- An impaired immune response
- Reduced ability of neutrophils to kill bacteria.

Cross-linking of collagen impairs wound healing. The formation of granulation tissue is delayed because of reduced fibroblast proliferation and migration. When fibroblasts are cultured on a medium containing 3-deoxyglucosone, a precursor of advanced glycation end products, their movement, proliferation, and secretion of collagen are impaired.

Wounds in non-diabetic pigs have been shown to be unaffected by a local hyperglycaemic environment, therefore wound healing in diabetes cannot be solely due to the increased osmolarity caused by hyperglycaemia. Tissue changes in cytokines and growth factors may be primarily responsible for the delayed healing in diabetic wounds.

Healing of oral wounds in the diabetic patient often has a better prognosis than healing of similar wounds in the foot. The oxygenation of centrally located structures is often superior and may explain the improved prognosis.

Are growth factors important in wound healing?

The absence of some growth factors in diabetic wounds may explain the delayed healing compared to non-diabetic wounds. In comparison with non-diabetic wounds there is an absence of insulin-like growth factor at the wound edge of diabetic ulcers and in dermal fibroblasts. Others point to the over-expression of tumour necrosis factor-α in diabetic ulcers.

References

20 Shyng YC, Devlin H, Sloan P. (2001) The effect of streptozotocin-induced experimental diabetes mellitus on calvarial defect healing and bone turnover in the rat. *Int J Oral Maxillofac Surg* **30**:70–4.

21 Hasegawa H, Ozawa S, Hashimoto K, Takeichi T, Ogawa T. (2008) Type 2 diabetes impairs implant osseointegration capacity in rats. *Int J Oral Maxillofac Implants* **23**:237–46.

22 Devlin H, Garland H, Sloan P. (1996) Healing of tooth extraction sockets in experimental diabetes mellitus. *J Oral Maxillofac Surg* **54**:1087–91.

23 Lu H, Kraut D, Gerstenfeld LC, Graves DT. (2003) Diabetes interferes with the bone formation by affecting the expression of transcription factors that regulate osteoblast differentiation. *Endocrinology* **144**:346–52.

24 Chrcanovic BR, Albrektsson T, Wennerberg A. (2014) Diabetes and oral implant failure: A systematic review. *J Dent Res* **93**:859–867.

25 Tawil G, Younan R, Azar P, Sleilati G. (2008) Conventional and advanced implant treatment in the type II diabetic patient: surgical protocol and long-term clinical results. *Int J Oral Maxillofac Implants* **23**:744–52.

Diabetes and severe infection

Diabetes type I has been recognized as a risk factor for severe infection with an increased risk of patient mortality. A recent study compared the bacterial colonization of deep neck infections in diabetic patients with those in non-diabetic patients and found that there was no difference in the percentage isolation of aerobic bacteria, but that anaerobic bacteria were more commonly isolated in non-diabetic patients.

There is little difference in the pathogenicity of the bacterial infection of patients with diabetes; they are prone to infection because of deficiencies in the body's defence mechanisms. This is the consequence of prolonged hyperglycaemia.

There are abnormalities in:
• Delayed migration of leukocytes
• Leukocyte phagocytosis is impaired.

Infection by antibiotic-resistant bacteria is rare if infections are acquired in the community. The most common infections in diabetes develop in the pharyngo-tonsillar region, urinary tracts, and skin.

Infection in diabetic patients can predispose them to ketoacidosis and hypoglycaemia.

In uncontrolled diabetes, severe head and neck infections include:
• Invasive external otitis. This is an infection of the external auditory canal and osteomyelitis of the temporal bone. Infection is caused by *Pseudomonas aeruginosa* and increasingly by meticillin-resistant *Staphylococcus aureus* (MRSA).
• Rhinocerebral mucormycosis characterized by tissue necrosis. This is an infection caused by the filamentous Zygomycetes fungi. The infection starts in the paranasal sinuses and can spread to the orbit and cranial cavity.

Diabetic foot ulceration

The major factors in the causation of diabetic foot ulceration are peripheral vascular disease and chronic peripheral neuropathy. The latter may involve sensory loss and loss of reflexes in the feet and dysesthesia. Patients are susceptible to foot injury, which can become infected and in extreme cases may require a limb amputation.

Diabetic foot ulcer treatment

This may involve
• Surgical debridement
• Antibiotic treatment accompanied by measures to remove the loading of the foot and to prevent pressure on the wound tissues
• Dressings
• Hyperbaric oxygen: This is where the patient inhales oxygen in a chamber at about 2.5 times higher pressure than normal. It increases the oxygen carrying capacity of the blood and counteracts the relative anoxia that can exist in the peripheral tissues of diabetic patients. The improved tissue perfusion improves collagen synthesis and angiogenesis.

Osteomyelitis of the jaw and diabetes

Uncontrolled diabetes is a risk factor for the development of osteomyelitis and can occur following a tooth extraction, trauma, or infections such as a dental abscess. Other major risk factors for osteomyelitis in the jaw include radiotherapy and intravenous bisphosphonates. Patients may complain of pain and swelling with a purulent discharge, and eventually exposure of necrotic bone

Osteomyelitis is usually classified into acute, sub-acute, and chronic conditions.

Acute osteomyelitis

Radiographic changes are usually minimal in the early acute stage. Diagnostic tests may involve:
- Technetium-99m bone scan, which will show increased uptake
- Raised erythrocyte sedimentation rate (ESR) and C-reactive protein
- Blood culture for the usual pathogens (such as S. aureus).

Treatment involves prolonged (4–6 weeks) antibiotic therapy that is active against S. aureus.

Chronic osteomyelitis

This chronic condition most commonly affects the mandible in elderly diabetic patient and may result from a dental abscess. By definition, the infection has a duration of longer than 6 weeks.

The low grade inflammation gives rise to fistulae and the exposure of necrotic bone (or sequestrum). The radiographic changes to the body of the mandible are seen as radiopaque sequestra surrounded by suppuration with ragged borders, often described as a moth-eaten appearance. Treatment involves surgical debridement and antibiotics.

Chronic active inflammation and extensive necrotic bone are present in the early healing stages of a tooth extraction socket of the diabetic rat. (See Fig. 7.2)

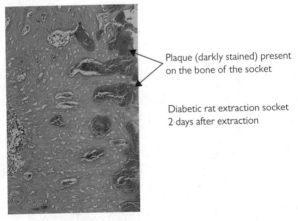

Plaque (darkly stained) present on the bone of the socket

Diabetic rat extraction socket 2 days after extraction

Fig. 7.2 Plaque present on rat alveolar bone surface 2 days after tooth extraction.

Summary

There is no evidence that giving well-controlled insulin-dependent diabetic patients prophylactic antibiotics prior to dental surgery is effective in reducing the rate of any subsequent infections. There is increasing concern about the inappropriate use of antibiotics causing antibiotic resistance and adverse patient reactions.

Summary recommendations

1. Amoxicillin can be given safely if infections develop.
2. Minor oral surgery can be performed on insulin-dependent diabetic patients within 2 hours of them having breakfast and their normal insulin injected dose.
3. Patients can recognize the symptoms of hypoglycaemia when meals are missed. They may become confused, sweaty, and have slurred speech. This can be treated by giving glucose (10–20 g) by mouth.
4. Hypoglylycaemia, causing unconsciousness, is an emergency which can be treated by injecting glucagon (adult dose of 1 mg) given intramuscularly (or by subcutaneous injection). Oral glucose can then be administered when the patient regains consciousness. If the patient fails to regain consciousness then they should be urgently transferred to the hospital.

Further reading

Lockhart P, Loven B, Brennan M, Fox P. (2007) The evidence base for the efficacy of antibiotic prophylaxis in dental practice. J Amer Dent Assoc [serial online]. **138**:458–7.

The respiratory system

The structure and function of the lungs 170
Control of respiratory exchange 172
Physiology of respiration 174
Localized airway obstruction 176
Obstructive sleep apnoea (OSA) 178
Lung disease 180
Anaesthesia and sedation 184

The structure and function of the lungs

The primary function of the lungs is to provide gas exchange by removing carbon dioxide produced by the tissues in metabolism and to deliver oxygen to the deoxygenated blood. However, of the inspired air, about 25% does not reach the alveoli and does not therefore play a role in gas exchange. This may seem an inefficient process, but it has the major advantage that large changes in alveolar concentration of gases are prevented during respiration.

What constitutes the non-respiratory conducting system?

Gas exchange does not occur at the trachea and bronchi. These conduct the gases to and from the alveoli and do not collapse during the respiratory pressure changes as they are reinforced by cartilage. The bronchi sub-divide into bronchioles (which do not contain cartilage).

The bronchioles are either:
- Terminal bronchioles (which conduct respiratory gases) and
- Respiratory bronchioles (which engage in respiratory exchange because they have alveoli budding from them).

How does gas exchange occur?

The respiratory lining is very thin and easily damaged.
- The lining of the alveolus is composed of mainly thin type I alveolar squamous epithelial cells that form the structure of the alveolar wall. Type II alveolar cells secrete pulmonary surfactant which reduces the surface tension of water and allows expansion of the alveoli during inspiration.
- Gas exchange occurs across the alveolar cells, the capillary endothelium, and their fused basal laminae.

Acute medical conditions preventing gas exchange
- Pulmonary oedema can occur following an MI and is the result of a rise in blood pressure in the left atrium. The effect is an increased amount of fluid passes from the alveolar capillaries into the interstitial space. It is characterized by breathlessness.
- Inflammation of the lungs (pneumonia) can impair gas exchange.
- Anaphylaxis is an allergic reaction and can result from taking medication, peanuts etc. in susceptible patients. The difficulty in breathing may be accompanied by a swelling of the tissues of the mouth and throat (which can further impair breathing).
- Inhalation of a foreign object.

Chronic medical conditions causing impaired gas exchange
- COPD
- Bronchiectasis where there are dilated bronchi, accompanied by frequent infections and coughing
- Anaemia may cause breathlessness during exertion
- Congestive heart failure
- Other conditions such as bronchial carcinoma where there is a small percentage of patients who present with breathlessness.

Physiological dead space

Ventilation and perfusion of the lungs must be matched to ensure maximally efficient gas exchange in the lungs. The physiological dead space includes both the air remaining in the respiratory conducting system and any alveoli that are not perfused by blood.

Clinical implications

In disease, if some alveoli are not perfused following blockage of a bronchiole by mucus, for example, then blood is redirected to the better ventilated areas of the lung.

The respiratory drive

The partial pressure of carbon dioxide (pCO_2) in the alveolus and the arterial blood is the key driver in the regulation of respiration. Changes in the partial pressure of oxygen (pO_2) in the alveolus play a lesser, but important, role.

- The arterial partial pressure of oxygen (PaO_2) is normally 75–100 mm Hg and the partial pressure of carbon dioxide ($PaCO_2$): 35–45 mm Hg.
- Over-ventilation causes little change in the arterial $PaO2$, but reduces the arterial $PaCO_2$. In those people who develop a panic attack, hyperventilation is an obvious sign. The immediate treatment is reassuring the patient and recommending slow, deep breathing exercises.
- Poor ventilation of some alveoli will cause an increase in the arterial $PaCO_2$ (and a respiratory acidosis).

Respiratory failure

Type 1 respiratory failure

This is characterized by low arterial blood oxygen (hypoxaemia) and a low or normal blood carbon dioxide. The cause is a failure in gas exchange. It may be accompanied by an increased rate or depth of respiration.

Type II respiratory failure

This is characterized by hypoxaemia (low PaO_2) and an elevated arterial carbon dioxide ($PaCO_2$ or hypercapnia). This ventilatory failure may be caused by sedatives, myopathy, or COPD. In COPD, the respiratory drive is from the hypoxia as the chemoreceptors become reset to accept the hypercapnia.

Control of respiratory exchange

Respiratory exchange in the lungs results in the oxygenation of the blood in the pulmonary artery and removal of carbon dioxide. Oxygen is absorbed from the alveolar gas and carbon dioxide diffuses from the blood into the alveolus. The breathing control mechanisms ensure that the partial pressure of alveolar carbon dioxide is inversely related to the rate of alveolar ventilation.

The pulmonary artery and vein

The pulmonary artery carries deoxygenated blood to the lungs from the right ventricle, while the pulmonary vein carries oxygenated blood from the lungs to the left ventricle. The pulmonary vessels have thin walls with lesser amounts of smooth muscle than would be expected in a similar-sized vessel from the systemic circulation. The pulmonary circulation is a lower pressure system than the systemic circulation.

Detection of lowered pH

Central chemoreceptors

Carbon dioxide, produced during metabolism, tends to cause an acidification of the bodily tissues. Respiration is one of the main mechanisms for controlling the acidity (or pH) of the blood; which has to be maintained within narrow limits (pH 7.35–7.45).

Increases in the pCO_2 of the cerebral arterial blood cause an increased diffusion of carbon dioxide into the extracellular fluid and cerebrospinal fluid. The equation below shows that the carbon dioxide reacts with water to form carbonic acid.

$$CO_2 + H_2O \leftrightarrow H_2CO_3 \leftrightarrow H^+ + HCO_3^-$$

An increased amount of carbon dioxide in the arterial blood forms carbonic acid in the cerebrospinal fluid. Because cerebrospinal fluid has less buffering capacity than blood, the change in pH is more profound and pH is reduced to lower than normal values. The altered pH is detected by the chemoreceptors and a respiratory response is activated.

Summary
The central chemoreceptors in the medulla detect when the pH of the cerebrospinal fluid is lowered (becomes more acidic). These activate the respiratory control centre in the medulla.

Peripheral chemoreceptors
These receptors are located in the aortic arch and at the junction of the internal and external carotid arteries. These receptors respond to a decreased arterial PaO_2, increased $PaCO_2$, and decreases in pH.

Summary
A reduced PO_2 in arterial blood (e.g. that can occur during mountaineering) is only sensed by peripheral chemoreceptors.

The medullary respiratory pattern generator

This is composed of a collection of cells (pre-Botzinger complex) which can generate pulsed firing patterns that give rise to a respiratory rhythm, and its production is not dependent on other sensory input.

Also in the medulla are:
- The dorsal respiratory group which is mainly associated with inspiration
- The ventral respiratory group which is mainly associated with expiration.

Both respiratory cell groups exhibit reciprocal inhibition during breathing. Other respiratory centres in the pons play a role; the apneustic centre (which has an excitatory function and increases the depth and duration of inspiration) and the pneumotaxic centre (which cyclically inhibits inspiration and regulates the amount of air intake).

This rhythm is modified depending on the input from the central and peripheral chemoreceptors, the cerebral cortex, and other brain centres.

Hering-Breuer reflex

This reflex prevents excessive dilation of the lung muscles by inhibiting deep inspiration.

Physiology of respiration

Spirometry

In these tests the patient is asked to expire air as quickly as possible. The amount of air exhaled in the first second is called FEV1, the forced expiratory volume in 1 s. Forced vital capacity (FVC) is the total amount of air exhaled during this test.

Significance of FEV1 and FVC in lung disease

Healthy individuals can expel, in a forced expiration, at least 70% of the FVC of the lungs in 1 s.

In health: FEV1 $> 0.7 \times$ FVC

However in chronic obstructive lung disease or asthma when the conducting airways may be blocked by mucus plugs, narrowing of the bronchi leads to a reduction in FEV1. The flow rate is reduced by the airway resistance.

In disease: FEV1 $< 0.7 \times$ FVC

Fig. 8.1 describes the changes in lung volume during normal breathing followed by a maximal inspiration and exhalation. A typical breathing frequency for a resting individual would be 15 breaths per minute. The total alveolar ventilation for the lungs is about 4–5 litres per minute. The total cardiac output is about 5 litres per minute. This gives a normal ventilation/perfusion (V/P) ratio of approximately 1.0 or thereabouts. In respiratory disease, the alveoli with decreased ventilation have a ventilation/perfusion ratio of less than 1.0.

There are regional differences in the ventilation–perfusion ratio in the lung. The ratio is high at the apex of the lung and lower at the lung base. With exercise, any regional differences tend to be reduced.

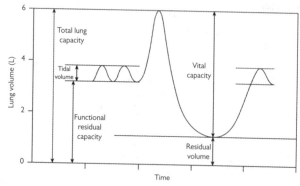

Fig. 8.1 Changes in lung volume during respiration.

Anatomic dead space (ADS)

During normal breathing, one breath of inspiration (or tidal volume), consists of about 500 ml. Part of this volume does not take part in gas exchange and is therefore called the dead space. This fraction remains in the conducting airways and consists of about 150 ml. The remaining 350 ml forms the alveolar gas which takes part in gas exchange.

In COPD, there are some areas of the lung which are not ventilated perhaps because the airways are occluded with mucus. In this situation, if the alveolus continues to be perfused there is an increased volume that is not participating in gas exchange. The total volume of air that does not participate in gas exchange includes poorly perfused and unventilated alveoli in addition to the anatomical space and is called the physiological dead space.

After a forced expiration in a patient with emphysema, the residual volume (the volume remaining in the lungs) is increased. The peripheral airways collapse during forced expiration because their poor supporting elastic tissue cannot resist the greater than atmospheric pressure. This impedes the airflow and leaves a considerable amount of gas remaining in the lung. This can give an appearance of an overinflated, barrel chest to the patient.

Functional residual capacity (FRC)

This is the volume of gas which remains in the lungs after an unforced expiration. Measurement of functional residual capacity can be undertaken using the helium dilution technique.

Summary
- Spirometry is a very useful technique in assessing the severity of COPD.
- COPD is diagnosed if FEV1 <80% predicted and FEV1/FVC <0.7 (70%).
- The severity of the airway obstruction is indicated by FEV1. In mild obstruction, FEV1 is between 50–80%. Severely affected patients have a FEV1 ranging from 30 to 49% that of healthy individuals and those who are very severely affected have a FEV1 <30%.

Localized airway obstruction

Partial obstruction of the airway results in a reduced ability for gas exchange to take place in the lungs. With upper airway obstruction, the patient has a loud, harsh-sounding stridor as they attempt to breathe, often using their accessory muscles of respiration. With complete obstruction, hypoxia is rapid and will be fatal.

The patient may seem confused and agitated as a result of the hypoxaemia and raised carbon dioxide concentration in the blood. Cyanosis is a late sign in the obstructed airway,

Causes of upper airway obstruction

- Maxillofacial injury may cause airway obstruction. This may also be accentuated by involvement of head injuries and a reduced level of consciousness.
- A squamous cell carcinoma of the larynx may cause a narrowing of the airway and significantly reduce airflow.
- A dentist may be luting a crown or other restoration in the mouth when it falls from their fingers and ends by obstructing the larynx. This can be avoided by placing gauze on the dorsum of the patient's tongue and around the tooth. In the first instance, the Heimlich manoeuvre may be used to dislodge the foreign object. Back blows and encouragement to cough may also be used.

Immediate treatment

The airway should be checked and expert assistance requested. If available, patients should receive supplemental oxygen with an oxygen mask (at a rate of 15 litres/min) and be placed in the recovery position with their face directed towards the ground. The UK resuscitation guidelines can be found at https://www.resus.org.uk/resuscitation-guidelines/adult-basic-life-support-and-automated-external-defibrillation/#foreign

Bronchial obstruction

Bronchial obstruction may result from aspiration of a small object such as a peanut. Usually the object lodges in the right main bronchus because this is wider and orientated more vertically than the left bronchus.

A normal cough reflex has a sensory component relayed by the superior laryngeal nerve with the motor response transmitted via the recurrent laryngeal nerve.

The absence of a protective cough reflex can give rise to silent aspiration. The result is that food and/or liquid pass through the patient's vocal cords into the lungs without arousing any suspicion amongst nursing staff that this has occurred. Those patient groups at particular risk include those with neurodegenerative conditions and stroke. In these conditions, patients are often unable to swallow and the continuous drooling of saliva is common. It is unproven whether the pathogenic bacteria present in periodontal disease may be aspirated and cause pneumonia following acute stroke.

Gastroesophageal reflux disease (GORD)

GORD and COPD commonly occur together. Both conditions may have a similar aetiology, tobacco smoking. Nicotine may induce a relaxation of the lower oesophageal sphincter. The co-occurrence of these conditions may increase the risk that there is aspiration into the lung of very small quantities of gastric contents. This may result in an increased frequency of acute exacerbations of COPD. The detection of gastric pepsin in pulmonary secretions would suggest the micro-aspiration of stomach contents.

Histamine2-receptor antagonists and proton pump inhibitor (PPI) therapy are successful in reducing the frequency of exacerbations of COPD in patients with GORD.

Inhalation of dentures and fixed partial dentures

Inhalation of dentures is not common, but impaction in the oesophagus occurs more frequently. It occurs more frequently in those who are alcohol and drug abusers and if the dentures are very small and retained poorly in the patient's mouth, this will also increase the likelihood of them being swallowed.

General anaesthesia involves an absence of laryngeal reflexes and a throat pack is used to protect the airway. Prior to its removal, any loose pieces of tissue, other debris, and tooth fragments in the oral cavity should be removed.

Minimizing the risk of inhalation during dental procedures

The use of a rubber dam is mandatory during endodontic procedures. It is a rubber sheet which has perforations through which the teeth can be accessed, while retracting the other oral tissues. The rubber dam is held in place on the teeth with clamps, elastic ligatures, or floss.

When handling crowns and fixed partial dentures in the patient's mouth:
• Have the patient seated in an upright position
• Place a gauze pack behind the teeth to protect the airway
• Tie floss around the fixed partial denture so that if it is dropped it can be easily retrieved from the floor of the patient's mouth.

The consequences of blocking an airway due to the inhalation of a foreign object or the presence of an obstructive neoplasm are to cause hypoxia and atelectasis, where alveolar air is absorbed resulting in collapse of that part of the lung. Other complications include pneumonia.

Obstructive sleep apnoea (OSA)

OSA is a very common condition that can be caused by a narrowing of the oro-pharyngeal airway, resulting in obstruction of the airway during sleep. If the cessation of breathing is for more than 10 seconds and occurs more than 10 times per hour during sleep, then it has clinically significant consequences. There is a reduction in the arterial pO2 level which triggers a waking response. The patient with OSA wakes frequently during the night, with the result that they are tired during the following day. Tiredness during the day results in a higher risk of motoring accidents, a general deterioration in the quality of the patient's life, and a disturbance in a partner's sleeping pattern.

Middle-aged, overweight individuals are especially affected, but the condition is underdiagnosed. Screening questionnaires are useful, e.g. Epworth sleepiness score. The diagnosis of OSA is expensive and confined to specialist centres. Obese patients with an enlarged neck may be at increased risk of OSA; the adipose tissue in the neck may narrow the airway.

Overnight pulse oximetry is often used as a first-line screening tool. This is a pulse/oxygen saturation sensor that the patient wears in their home overnight. If the result of this investigation is not diagnostic, then in-laboratory polysomnography is usually used.

Aetiology

A number of theories have been suggested for the upper airway blockage:
1. One theory involves local changes in the pharyngeal tissues. These include impairment of the upper airway muscle function and coordination caused by the intermittent hypoxia during OSA. The soft palate may also become oedematous following trauma caused by snoring.
2. It has been suggested that the aetiology of OSA is due to fluid redistribution during sleep. It is hypothesized that fluid accumulates in the legs during the day and then is gradually redistributed to the neck region when the patient lies down to go to sleep.

Risk factors

Obstructive sleep apnoea is associated with:
- Obesity
- Excessive cigarette smoking and alcohol consumption
- Hypertension, especially in those with drug resistance.

Changes occurring during obstructive sleep apnoea

Short-term changes

There is a short hypoxaemia, which returns to normal when the patient resumes normal breathing. Patients complain of being drowsy during the day, and their snoring can affect the sleeping pattern of partners.

Long-term changes

Obesity is strongly associated with OSA and insulin resistance. However, some studies hypothesize that OSA may have an additional deleterious effect on increasing insulin resistance.

There is increased sympathetic activity in OSA causing an increased peripheral resistance. This is caused by the effects of repeated hypoxia and hypercapnia on the autonomic nervous system. OSA is therefore associated with an increased risk of systemic hypertension, ventricular hypertrophy, and coronary artery disease. Increased blood and urinary concentrations of catecholamines have been found in patients with OSA.

Treatment of sleep apnoea

Mandibular advancement prostheses

These intra-oral appliances hold the mandible and tongue in a forward position to create space posteriorly in the pharynx. Mild effects are noted in the occlusion of long-term wearers of oral OSA prostheses; overbite and overjet are reduced by about 1 mm. Though these changes are mild, the occlusion of these patients should be monitored by regular dental review. The occlusal changes occur due to the force generated on the anterior teeth by the mandible attempting to return to its normal position.

The prostheses are worn during sleep. This treatment is effective in treating mild and moderate OSA.

Continuous positive airway pressure (CPAP)

CPAP is a device which applies mild air pressure through a mask which fits over the patient's nose and mouth. This increased air pressure prevents the airway from becoming blocked. It is effective in treating the more severely affected patients with OSA.

Beneficial effect of CPAP and mandibular advancement prostheses

There is evidence that mandibular advancement prostheses and CPAP have beneficial effects on reducing blood pressure and improving the alertness of sufferers experienced during the day. CPAP has been shown to result in reduced insulin resistance.

Lung disease

Chronic obstructive pulmonary disease (COPD)

This is mainly caused by smoking and all health professionals should discourage patients from smoking. It is a common disease and an important cause of mortality. Patients are increasingly breathless and commonly have a productive cough. Patients with COPD are rarely aged less than 35 years of age, whereas those affected by asthma are often young.

Clinical presentation

The term 'chronic obstructive pulmonary disease' includes chronic bronchitis and emphysema.

Emphysema

With emphysema there is destruction of the alveolar walls. The air spaces distal to the terminal bronchioles are enlarged, which is visible using a CT scan. Because of the diminished gas exchange, the affected patients may have shortness of breath (dyspnea) and a chronic cough. Following smoking over the long-term, emphysema may be caused by a series of different pathogenic events:

- Protease-anti-protease imbalance.
- Elastases released by neutrophils and macrophages remove the lung collagen and elastin. The breakdown products encourage further inflammation, resulting in alveolar destruction.
- Matrix metalloproteinases (MMPs) are proteolytic enzymes which are increased in the airways of COPD patients and may breakdown pulmonary extracellular matrix.

Chronic bronchitis

With chronic bronchitis, patients have a cough which lasts at least 3 months a year for more than 2 years. The bronchi become inflamed as a result of cigarette smoking, excess mucus is produced, and the airways become narrowed.

Most patients with COPD function within a spectrum exemplified by two extremes groups. At one end of the spectrum are those with a high ventilatory effort resulting in a normal pCO_2 and at the other end are cyanotic patients with an increased pCO_2

COPD is characterized by airway obstruction, over-inflation of the lungs and a poor tolerance to exercise.

Severe complications of COPD include:

- Pulmonary hypertension
- Enlargement of the right side of the heart and heart failure
- Lung cancer (as a result of the cigarette smoking)
- Respiratory infections. (It is recommended that all patients receive an annual flu vaccination).

Chronic bronchitis may be treated with antibiotics and bronchodilator drugs.

Summary

There are several points of particular relevance to the dentist in treating patients with COPD

- Patients with COPD may prefer to be treated sitting upright to assist in their breathing.
- All health personnel should advise smoking cessation. Dry mouth may result from continual mouth breathing and the side effect of nicotine replacement therapy drugs.
- There is no conclusive evidence of chronic periodontitis playing a major role in causing acute exacerbations of COPD.
- There is an increased risk of oropharyngeal candidiasis in those taking inhaled corticosteroids. Following inhaler use, patients should rinse out their mouth.

Lung cancer

Symptoms

Symptoms may include haemoptysis (coughing up blood) and a persistent cough lasting over 3 weeks. Chest pain is a late symptom. Patients may have difficulty breathing and unexplained weight loss. Dentists who suspect patients may have lung cancer should encourage early general medical practitioner review and respiratory clinic referral.

Epidemiology

This is a disease with a poor survival rate, mainly because the majority of patients present with an advanced stage of the disease. However, over 80% of early stage lung cancer in high risk individuals can be detected using low-dose CT, thus providing a better chance of survival.

An internet based questionnaire can be used to provide an individual's lung cancer risk in the next 5 years (see htttp://www.MylungRisk.org). It was developed by the University of Liverpool, Cancer Research Centre and is based on those risk factors that increase the risk of lung cancer (i.e. age, gender, smoking duration, family history of lung cancer, previous history of pneumonia, previous diagnosis of cancer, and exposure to asbestos).

Asthma

In asthma there is a variable amount of airway obstruction and narrowing of the lumen due to inflammation. In asthma, the mucous is especially viscous. The patient may be taking inhaled corticosteroids and β2-adrenergic agonists. There are rarely systemic side-effects from the inhaled steroid.

Clinical dental relevance

The main potential concern is the increased rate of caries that can result from the dry mouth brought on by using β2-adrenergic agonists. Regular dental check-ups are essential, with the use of topical fluoride supplements where necessary. Inhaled oral steroids are associated with an increased risk of candidiasis and patients are encouraged to rinse out their mouths with water following use of the inhaler.

Asthma and caries

In a systematic review and meta-analysis, patients with asthma were found to have a significantly increased risk of caries[1]. The risk is approximately doubled. The reason for this may be due to the reduced saliva flow produced by β2-adrenergic agonists and an increased number of *Streptococcus mutans* in the saliva of asthmatics. β2-adrenergic stimulation of the salivary glands produces a thick saliva. Inhaler use does not produce an acidogenic response that takes the plaque pH below 5.5, the critical pH at which enamel begins to dissolve.

Recognizing an asthma attack in adults

An asthma attack can be brought on by the stress of attending a dentist. Acute severe asthma is characterized by an inability to complete sentences, tachycardia (an abnormally fast resting heart rate), and tachypnea (abnormally rapid breathing). Those suffering from a life-threatening asthma attack often appear exhausted with poor respiratory effort and an altered level of consciousness[2].

Call for help from the emergency services early. Many deaths from asthma are preventable and delay and failure to recognize the severity of an attack can be fatal. Whilst waiting for the ambulance to arrive the dentist should administer inhaled β2-adrenergic agonists, such as salbutamol which is often prescribed to the patient as a blue Ventolin® metered dose inhaler. Patients should be encouraged to take 4 puffs via a spacer initially, followed by a further 2 puffs every 2 minutes according to response up to a maximum of 10 puffs. It is important to have a calm, measured approach. The dentist should also administer oxygen (15 litres/min) to maintain the patient's oxygen saturations (SpO2) at 94–98%. Even if the patient has a good response to the treatment measures delivered, they should be reviewed by a medical doctor the same day. (➔ See Table 8.1)

Inhalation sedation in asthma

For the well-controlled asthmatic child, inhalation sedation is not contraindicated. However, it is usually contraindicated in those children with severe asthma because nitrous oxide can irritate the airway.

Preventive dentistry

In patients where asthma has required hospitalization, fluoride varnish application to the teeth to prevent tooth decay may be contraindicated.

Allergy to aspirin

Asthmatic children have an increased prevalence of allergy to aspirin and a paediatric form of paracetamol is recommended instead.

Table 8.1 Clinical implications

Summary	Clinical implication
Aspirin	Can precipitate an asthma attack.
Inhaled Steroid	Can cause an increased risk of oral candidiasis. This may require antifungal agents to be prescribed.
Mouth breathing	Can predispose to gingivitis. Reinforce oral hygiene instruction.
Smoking	All asthmatics should avoid smoking.

Can the generating of aerosols in dental surgeries cause disease?

Aerosols are frequently generated by dentists using high speed dental turbines and ultrasonic scaling procedures. Ultrasonic scalers remove plaque from the tooth surface using cavitation in the water spray that cools the vibrating tip. There is an increased risk of infection with *Mycobacterium tuberculosis* that is greater than that for the general population[3].

Cross-infection control measure to protect against aerosol exposure

- Face masks that provide an effective filter of air in the surgery
- Efficient aspiration of saliva and water coolant by the assistant
- If the patient rinses their mouth with an antiseptic before scaling then there is a reduced bacterial count in the aerosol produced.

Inhalation of particles of less than 2.5 μm can result in their passage to the alveoli. Chronic exposure by dental workers to aerosol debris resulting from tooth preparation procedures should be avoided.

References

1   Alavaikko S, Jaakkola MS, Tjäderhane L, Jaakkola JJ. (2011) Asthma and caries: a systematic review and meta-analysis. *Am J Epidemiol* **174**:631–41.
2   The British Thoracic Society management of acute asthma guidelines at https://www.britthoracic.org.uk/document-library/clinical-information/asthma/btssign-asthma-guideline-2012/
3   Bennett AM, Fulford MR, Walker JT, Bradshaw DJ, Martin MV, Marsh PD (2000) Microbial aerosols in general dental practice. *Br Dent J*. **189**:664–7.

Anaesthesia and sedation

To control anxiety and pain for some dental procedures, conscious sedation or general anaesthesia may be needed. The clinician should fully assess the case and choose the simplest and safest technique that is likely to be effective.

General anaesthesia

The American Society of Anesthesiologists approved the following classification of patients (see ASA Relative Value Guide®). (➔ See Table 8.2)

Patients with cardiovascular or lung disease undergoing a general anaesthetic require careful pre-operative assessment with the patient treated in hospital.

Inhalational sedation

This sedation technique is especially valuable in sedating anxious children, who may not respond well to benzodiazepines. If treated with benzodiazepines, children are more likely to undergo an adverse, paradoxical reaction (about 1.4%). This is characterized by aggression, agitation, disorientation, and restlessness. Paradoxical reactions are treated by ensuring the patient has an adequate airway and circulation, with reversal of the benzodiazepine sedation with flumazenil.

Nitrous oxide has a sedative action. The technique of inhalation sedation involves the administration of a gas mixture of oxygen and nitrous oxide through a nasal mask. In this technique, the patient does not lose consciousness, but feels relaxed and able to cooperate with the dentist. Distraction of the child is an important part of the technique. Nitrous oxide sedation is the first choice for conscious sedation in children (over 4 years)[4].

Table 8.2 ASA Classifications

ASA classification	Definition
ASA I	Healthy patient
ASA II	Mild disease present, e.g. mild lung disease
ASA III	Severe systemic disease present, e.g. poorly controlled diabetes
ASA IV	Severe disease that threatens life, e.g. recent myocardial infarction
ASA V	Patient is moribund and will not survive without the operation
ASA VI	Patient is brain-dead

Actions of nitrous oxide

Nitrous oxide appears to have multiple mechanisms of action to achieve its varied properties:

- Analgesic effect by stimulating neuronal release of endogenous opioid peptides
- Anxiolytic effect by activating the inhibitory neurotransmitter, GABA in a similar way to benzodiazepines
- Anaesthetic effect by inhibiting the normally CNS excitatory influence of NMDA (N-methyl-D-aspartate glutamate)[5].

Inhalation sedation technique

100% oxygen can be administered at any time, if needed. Inhalation sedation commences by using 100% oxygen (at a flow rate of 4 litres/min for children). The patient is instructed to breathe through the nose and semi-hypnotic suggestions are given. The concentration of nitrous oxide is increased gradually to 10% after 1 minute and to eventually about 30–50% depending on the patient's need. The concentration of inhaled nitrous oxide must not exceed 70%. Clinical monitoring of the patient is essential. At this concentration, nitrous oxide has little analgesic action so local anaesthetic should be administered when undertaking dental treatment. When the dental procedures have finished, the child is given 100% oxygen for a few minutes. Scavenging of gases is essential to avoid risks to the dental team. Pulse oximetry is not required for inhalation sedation. Scavenging equipment is needed to ensure safety for the operating room staff.

Contraindications to inhalation sedation

Anxious children or adults who are in ASA I or II (➔ See Table 8.2) can be given conscious sedation in general dental practice and do not require referral to hospital. Those in higher categories should be referred for hospital treatment. There are few contraindications to this procedure, especially if the administration of the nitrous oxide is for less than 10–15 minutes. There is an increased incidence of nausea and vomiting with longer procedures. Fasting rules vary across Europe, but one guideline recommends that no solid foods or milk are given less than 4 hours before sedation[6]. (EAPD guidelines on sedation in paediatric dentistry. 2003). Children under school age may drink sugar containing clear liquids up to 2 hours before treatment in order to avoid low blood sugar.

Specific contraindications to inhalation sedation include patients with nasal blockage after a cold or tonsillitis, porphyria, psychosis, or those patients taking bleomycin chemotherapy.

References

[4] IACSD (Intercollegiate Advisory Committee for Sedation in Dentistry) 2015. Standards for Conscious Sedation in the Provision of Dental Care. London: RCS Publications.

[5] Emmanouil DE, Quock RM. (2007). Advances in understanding the actions of nitrous oxide. *Anesthesia Progress* 54, 9–18.

[6] Hallonsten AL, Jensen B, Raadal M, Veerkamp J, Hosey MT, Poulsen S. (2015). EAPD guidelines on sedation in paediatric dentistry. http://www.eapd.eu/8B927172.en.aspx

Chapter 9

Heart and blood supply

Function of the heart 188
Control of heart contraction 190
Control of cardiovascular system 194
Atherosclerosis 196
Heart failure 198
Infections and the heart 202
Stroke (cerebrovascular accident or CVA) 204

Function of the heart

The heart has 4 chambers.

- **Right atrium** receives blood from superior and inferior vena cava
- Blood then passes through the tricuspid value (right AV valve) into the right ventricle
- **Right ventricle** pumps blood to the lungs through pulmonary valves via pulmonary arteries
- **Left atrium** receives blood from pulmonary veins and it then passes through the mitral valve (left AV valve) into
- **Left ventricle** which pumps blood to general circulation through the aortic valve to the aorta.

The pump action of the heart at rest takes around 1 second, ejecting around 70 mL (the stroke volume) into the aorta. Typically 70 beats/minute gives a cardiac output of 4,900 mL of blood (cardiac output = rate × stroke volume).

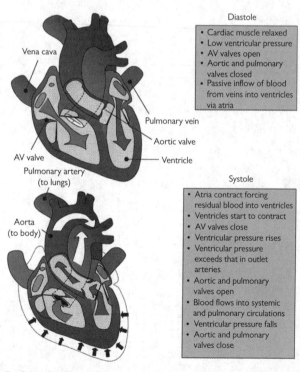

Diastole
- Cardiac muscle relaxed
- Low ventricular pressure
- AV valves open
- Aortic and pulmonary valves closed
- Passive inflow of blood from veins into ventricles via atria

Vena cava

Pulmonary vein

Aortic valve

AV valve

Ventricle

Pulmonary artery (to lungs)

Aorta (to body)

Systole
- Atria contract forcing residual blood into ventricles
- Ventricles start to contract
- AV valves close
- Ventricular pressure rises
- Ventricular pressure exceeds that in outlet arteries
- Aortic and pulmonary valves open
- Blood flows into systemic and pulmonary circulations
- Ventricular pressure falls
- Aortic and pulmonary valves close

Fig. 9.1 The cardiac cycle. Reproduced with permission from *Oxford Handbook of Medical Sciences*, with permission from Oxford University Press.

The myocardium is made up of specialized branching cardiac muscle cells, each with one nucleus and many mitochondria. Each cardiac muscle cell has specialized connections (intercalated discs) which contain anchoring junctions (desmosomes) and electrical junctions (gap junctions) which allow action potentials to pass directly from cell to cell allowing the myocardium to act like a single cell and a wave of electrical potential to result in a synchronized heart contraction. (➜ See Fig. 9.1 and Table 9.1.)

Heart valves

The correct functioning of the heart valves is crucial to the effective functioning of the heart. They stop backflow in the system and ensure forward propulsion of the blood. Heart failure develops if valve function is seriously impaired. Impairment takes two forms:

- Regurgitation (incompetence and backflow) caused by endocarditis, valve prolapse, or valve disease
- Stenosis (flow is impeded) caused by rheumatic fever, atherosclerosis, congenital heart disease, or calcification.

Investigations—auscultation for heart murmur, ECG.
Treatment—valvoplasty or valve replacement.

Table 9.1 The cardiac cycle

Stage	Activity	ECG
Diastole	Heart muscle relaxes	P wave
	Ventricle pressure ↓	
	Atrio-ventricular valves open	
	Pulmonary and aortic valves are closed	
	Passive filling from circulation via atria into ventricles	
Systole	Atria contract	QRS complex
	Ventricles start to contract	T-wave
	Atrio-ventricular valves close	Heart sound 1 = AV values closing
	Ventricle pressure ↑	
	Pulmonary and aortic valves open	Heart sound 2 = aortic & pulmonary valves closing
	Ejection into systemic circulation (~50ml remains—ESV)	
	Ventricle pressure ↓	
	Pulmonary and aortic valves close	

ESV = end systolic volume

Control of heart contraction

A patch of specialized cells on the posterior wall of the right atrium known as the sinoatrial node (SA node) originates an impulse that spreads through the heart as a wave of depolarization. (➔ See Fig. 9.2). The rate of firing of the SA node is moderated by autonomic nerves:
• Parasympathetic: reduces heart rate and contractility
• Sympathetic: increases heart rate and contractility.

Sympathetic stimulation also has an effect on the general circulation causing vasoconstriction of peripheral arteries (impeding blood flow and increasing peripheral resistance) and veins. Venous vasoconstriction makes the veins stiffer, increasing central venous pressure, reducing pooling, and aiding return of blood to the heart.

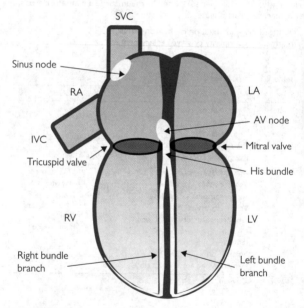

Fig. 9.2 The conducting system of the heart. Reproduced from Timperley, J., et al, *Pacemakers and ICDs*, 2007, with permission form Oxford University Press.

The sequence of events is:
1. SA (sinus) node fires.
2. Depolarization spreads from cell to cell across the atria.
3. Annulus fibrosus (band of connective tissue) stops spread to ventricles and isolates atria from ventricles except at the atrioventricular (AV) node.
4. Impulse is channelled to the AV node (small cells which slow the spread of the impulse). This delay allows time for atrial contraction to fill the ventricles.
5. Transmission of the signal down the wide cells (fast conducting) of the bundle of His and Purkinje fibres down the interventricular wall and along the inner surface of both ventricles.

In health this system ensures that only one electrical impulse is generated at any time and it travels in one direction ensuring a co-ordinated heart action.

The electrocardiogram (ECG)

This electrical activity in the heart can be detected as small voltage changes at the skin surface. Classically ECG readings are described as below. (➲ See Fig. 9.3.)

Cardiac output of approx. 4,900 mL per minute is achieved by the heart ejecting stroke volume of 70 mL and beating 70 times per minute (stroke volume × pulse rate).

Stroke volume is dependent on:
• Myocardial contractility (depends on Ca^{2+})
• Filling pressure from venous return
• Resistance to outflow through aorta.

Because the circulation is a closed system, cardiac output must be the same as venous return.

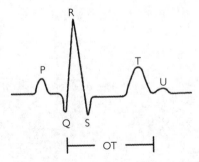

Fig. 9.3 Normal ECG. Reproduced with permission from *Applied Medicine and Surgery in Dentistry*, with permission from Oxford University Press.

Arrythmias

This process may be disrupted by an infarct and scarring in the cardiac tissue following a myocardial infarction (MI). SA node may be affected but usually other areas take over this role. AV node being affected may mean uncoupling of the co-ordination of sequential contraction of atria then ventricles (known as heart block). One-way transmission of the electrical impulse may be disturbed over part of the cardiac muscle. Management includes: artificial pacemaker, surgical ablation of a damaged area, and drugs.

Atrial fibrillation

This is a very rapid (300–600 per minute) and irregular contraction of the atria. Ventricular contraction is also abnormal as ventricular contraction is initiated for only some of the atrial contractions. Causes include MI, hypertension, hyperthyroidism, heart failure. There is a risk of thromboembolism. Management is with anticoagulants and drugs to slow atrial contractions (β blockers, Ca^{2+} channel blockers, digoxin).

Control of cardiovascular system

Control of cardiac output

According to Starling's law of the heart, the energy released during contraction depends of the initial fibre length. That is, the force of contraction is proportional to the end diastolic volume, which is dependent on the volume of blood returning to the heart. Greater stretch to the optimal allows more myosin cross-bridges to form and hence increases the force that can be generated. Because the circulation is a closed system cardiac output must be the same as venous return. However, the system can be adjusted by:

- Pooling in the venous circulation by dilating these vessels
- Increasing contractility of heart muscle by sympathetic stimulation.

Control of blood pressure (BP) (⊜ see also Chapter 6)

Baroreceptors in carotid sinus and aortic arch are sensitive to stretch in the vessel walls. A reduction in distension denotes a fall in mean arterial pressure (MAP). This triggers a reduction in stimulation via vagus and glossopharyngeal nerves to the autonomic centre in the medulla. Sympathetic stimulation increases heart rate and contractility and produces vasoconstriction of arterioles and veins. Hence cardiovascular pressure (CVP) rises. Parasympathetic stimulation contributes to slow the heart rate.

This process is vital in maintaining MAP and cerebral perfusion after blood loss. In addition, other mechanisms are brought in to restore blood volume.

- Sympathetic stimulation → renal arterioles constrict → renal perfusion ↓ → Na & water retained, urine output suppressed
- Sympathetic stimulation and ↓ MAP activate renin-angiotensin II → vasoconstriction
- Angiotensin II → aldosterone → increased renal Na reabsorption
- Angiotensin II & antidiuretic hormone (ADH) → thirst.

Hypertension is persistently raised BP (>140/90 mmHg) due to increased arteriolar resistance. Mostly this occurs with no identified cause (essential hypertension). Hypertension also occurs as a complication of renal disease or diabetes mellitus.

Clinical relevance

Patients taking antihypertensive drugs may experience postural hypotension and transient loss of consciousness if they get up quickly from a lying to a standing position.

Fainting (syncope)

This is a familiar event. The patient feels dizzy, weak, nauseous, is pale, with cold, clammy skin, and they may lose consciousness. Syncope occurs when cerebral blood flow and oxygenation fall below a critical value. Maintenance of cerebral perfusion has an intricate and complex feedback system. Baroreceptor reflexes are a key part of this and regulate BP mainly via increasing venous return and increasing heart rate. Powerful vasoconstriction and the peripheral muscle pump increase venous return. These efforts may be sufficient to ward off the threat of syncope but if not, then something triggers a sudden change from vasoconstriction and tachycardia to vasodilation and bradycardia. It used to be thought that stimulation of cardiac receptors was the trigger but some cerebral signal is more probable. The nucleus tractus solitarii of the brainstem triggers stimulation of the parasympathetic nervous system (vagal) reducing heart rate and contractility producing a decrease in cardiac output, large enough to result in a loss of consciousness. Simultaneous inhibition of the sympathetic nervous system produces vasodilation and a fall in BP. Predisposing factors are being upright for long periods, motionless, and warm; being dehydrated or emotionally stressed; and blood loss. Management of syncope is by placing the patient supine with legs raised to enable haemodynamic equilibrium and cerebral perfusion to be restored.

Response to sudden blood loss

In blood loss all the processes described to control BP work together to restore circulating blood volume. Arterial baroreceptors sense a reduction in BP and trigger the sympathetic nervous system to increase heart rate and contractility so that cardiac output is maintained. Sympathetic stimulation constricts venous capacitance vessels in skin and splanchnic arterial beds, to maintain BP. The constricted arterioles result in decreased capillary pressure. Since osmotic pressure remains unaltered in tissue fluid, the net result is a movement of fluid out of the interstitial space and into blood. The interstitial fluid loss is replaced within a few hours. The direct effect of reduced renal perfusion reduces urine production. The reduced arterial pressure and sympathetic stimulation activates the renin-angiotensin-aldosterone system resulting in further retention of sodium and water, helping restore blood volume. Bone marrow is stimulated to replace the lost cells and releases immature reticulocytes into circulation. Replacement of erythrocytes can take several weeks. The response to blood loss is proportional to the amount lost. Severe blood loss, in excess of 40% of the total volume, will result in irreversible 'shock' if a blood transfusion is not given within the first hour of trauma (golden hour). Without this, prolonged tissue ischaemia, build-up of acidity and toxins leads to multi-organ failure.

Atherosclerosis

Atherosclerosis is a complex disease process characterized by the formation of fatty plaques in the walls of arteries, leading to impaired circulation. Plaques form at areas of turbulent flow, at bends and branching points. While such plaques start forming in most of us from an early age they are much more common in association with risk factors: diabetes; smoking; hypertension; high lipid diet; genetic predisposition; being male. Cholesterol and lipids accumulate in the intimal surface of arterial walls forming atheromatous plaques. The sequence of events is:

1. Erosion/dysfunction of the endothelium including loss of nitric oxide protective effects. These cells become activated, expressing a variety of adhesion molecules which attract monocytes which migrate beneath the endothelium and differentiate into macrophages. Endothelial erosion exposes sub-endothelium which attracts platelets forming micro-thrombi.

2. An inflammatory process involving T lymphocytes, macrophages, and platelets occurs. In response, local smooth muscle cells proliferate and migrate into the intima. These are non-contractile and secretory generating extracellular matrix which stabilizes the plaque.

3. Lipids (LDL) accumulate and are oxidized. These are phagocytosed by macrophages (foam cells) and when these die they release their lipid into the plaque. As the plaque matures inflammation resolves and calcification may also occur. The atheromatous plaque may stabilize at this point or may go onto:
   • Reduce blood flow distal to the plaque
   • Rupture and resolve spontaneously
   • Rupture and form a clot (platelet-fibrin thrombus) on its surface which may then break up and travel in the circulation, forming a thromboembolus
   • Produce thinning and weakening of the vessel wall and ballooning out as an aneurysm.

Coronary arteries are particularly susceptible to atherosclerosis for several reasons:
• Flow is disturbed by the contracting heart muscle.
• Coronary arteries are very branched and tortuous.
• There is little collateral circulation.

The three major coronary arteries are the:
• Left anterior descending artery
• Left circumflex artery
• Right coronary artery.

Most people with angina have blockages in one or more of these arteries and/or their branches.
• Myocardial ischaemia (insufficient blood in the heart muscle) results when the narrow arteries do not allow enough blood to reach the heart during periods of physical or emotional stress. This lack of blood will trigger an episode of angina.

Angina

Angina is a short lasting chest pain caused by ischaemia in heart muscle and which stops on resting or with glyceryl trinitrate (GTN). GTN acts to relax smooth muscle cells and produce vasodilation.

Angina is categorized as:

Stable angina
- Symptoms are brought on by exercise or stress
- Usually only last a few minutes
- Can be improved by taking GTN.

Unstable angina
- Symptoms develop without any trigger
- May last longer than 5 minutes
- May persist even when resting
- May not respond to treatment with GTN.

Myocardial infarction (MI)

Signs and symptoms
- Persistent severe crushing pain which may radiate to left mandible, arm, neck
- Tightness of chest
- Breathlessness
- Nausea and vomiting
- Loss of consciousness
- Weak or irregular pulse.

Atypical presentation (e.g. MI without chest pain) is more likely in females, diabetics, and older adults.

Emergency management of MI
- Give GTN
- Call ambulance
- If not allergic, give 300 mg aspirin to be crushed intra-orally (tell ambulance crew)
- Reassure the patient and allow patient to rest in comfortable position
- Give oxygen (if available, give nitrous oxide and oxygen 50:50)
- Monitor the patient.

Clinical relevance

Dental treatment should be deferred in unstable or newly diagnosed angina. After MI any elective procedures are best delayed for a year. Appointments should be kept short, preferably avoid mornings and every effort should be made to limit discomfort and anxiety. The dentist should liaise closely with the physician. Prophylactic GTN may be advised and careful monitoring may be recommended.

Heart failure

Cardiac failure occurs when the heart is unable to maintain sufficient cardiac output to meet the demands of the body. It is very common, especially in older adults. Common causes include: ischaemic heart disease, hypertension, and COPD. The sequence of events following MI and damage to part of the myocardium might be:

1. Cardiac output reduces
2. BP reduces & is detected by baroreceptors and in reduced kidney blood flow
3. Baroreceptors trigger sympathetic stimulation producing:
   • ↑Heart rate
   • ↑Blood volume
   • ↑Vascular resistance/tone
4. Cardiac output is restored

This is a short-term fix for the problem but longer term a vicious spiral develops.

• The increased demand on the heart stimulates the ventricle walls to thicken thus increasing the force of contraction but this has the effect of reducing the volume of the ventricles, reducing stroke volume.
• Reduced renal perfusion triggers the renin–angiotensin–aldosterone system and produces blood pooling in the periphery and ↑ CVP. While this should increase the force of contraction, this is already increased and further demand produces overload.

Clinical presentation

This is of fatigue, breathlessness, and oedema. If the failure is mainly affecting the left side of the heart, the main features are blood damming back in the pulmonary circulation resulting in pulmonary oedema, cyanosis, and dyspnoea. If the failure is mainly affecting the right side of the heart, congestion is in the systemic side especially affecting the liver, kidney, and GI tract. Pressure in the portal circulation is raised, and ascites and peripheral oedema result.

Management

By treatment of the cause and the symptoms. Various drugs may be used. (See Table 9.2.) Pacemaker, implantable cardiac defibrillator, or heart transplant may be required.

Clinical relevance

Heart failure should be managed before any dental treatment is attempted.

Early morning appointments are best avoided as cardiac events are most likely then due to high levels of endogenous adrenaline. Patients with dyspnoea should be treated sitting upright. Bupivacaine should be avoided. Adrenaline should not be used for gingival retraction and in local anaesthesia (LA) should be limited to 2 cartridges. Anxiety and pain may precipitate arrhythmia or angina so must be managed well. Sedation may be possible but GA requires great care and there is an increased risk of venous thrombosis and pulmonary embolus.

Table 9.2 Drugs commonly used to manage heart failure

Problem	Drug	Action
Volume overload	Diuretics e.g. furosemide, bumetanide	Loss of fluid from circulation
Volume overload	ACE inhibitors*, e.g. ramipril, captopril Angiotensin receptor blockers (ARB), e.g. candesartan, losartan Aldosterone antagonists, e.g. spironolactone, eplerenone	Produce vasodilation and increase cardiac contractility
Sympathetic overstimulation	β blockers, e.g. bisoprolol, carvedilol	Inhibits β adrenergic receptors to slow the heart and reduce BP
Insufficient contractility	Cardiac glycosides e.g. digoxin	Increased contractility Slows heart Improves rhythm
Resistance overload	Organic nitrates e.g. isosorbide mononitrate	Vaso/veno dilation

*Renin (from kidney) converts angiotensinogen to angiotensin I, which is converted in the lungs by angiotensin converting enzyme (ACE) to angiotensin II. Angiotensin II stimulates the adrenal cortex to produce aldosterone which induces peripheral vasoconstriction. Aldosterone activates the pump in the distal renal tubule leading to reabsorption of sodium and water from urine, in exchange for potassium and hydrogen ions. ACE inhibitors inhibit this process.

Implanted devices

Cardiovascular implantable electronic devices (CIED) are common treatments for arrhythmias. These include pacemakers and automatic defibrillators. Adrenaline use should be limited in such patients to a maximum of 2 cartridges of adrenaline containing LA and no use of adrenaline in gingival retraction. Another hazard is electromagnetic interference. So MRI scans, electrosurgery, and diathermy should not be used. Possible interference may occur with electric pulp tester, apex locators, and ultrasonic scalers. Such items should be kept at least 30 cm away from the implant and with any interference, further use should cease.

Heart transplant

Patients planned for heart transplant should have careful pre-operative dental assessment to eliminate any oral sources of infection and to establish good oral self-care regime. No dental treatment should be undertaken for the first 6 months following the transplant.

Commonly used drugs

Table 9.3 lists some complication and interactions for drugs commonly used for cardiovascular conditions. Close liaison with the patient's physician is crucial.

Table 9.3 Dental relevance of drugs commonly prescribed for cardio-vascular disease

Drug type, drug action, and examples	Dental relevance
Beta blockers *Action*: to inhibit sympathetic effects on CVS *Examples*: atenolol, propranolol, sotalol	• Limit adrenaline containing LA to 2 cartridges (to avoid uncompensated BP rise) • Dry mouth and lichenoid reactions are possible

ACE Inhibitors
Action: to inhibit the conversion of angiotensin I to angiotensin II.
Examples: ramipril, lisinopril
	• Possible side-effects are:
	  • Dry mouth
	  • Burning mouth
	  • Oral ulceration
	  • Angioedema
	  • Lichenoid reaction
	• Possible drug interaction with NSAIDs

Statins *Action*: to reduce LDL-cholesterol levels which in turn reduces risks of MI and CVA *Examples*: simvastatin, atorvastatin	• Drug interaction with azole antifungals (e.g. miconazole, fluconazole) • Drug interaction with macrolide antibiotics (e.g. erythromycin) • Potentially serious myopathy may occur
Vitamin K antagonist anti-coagulants *Action*: to prevent thrombus formation and strokes *Examples*: warfarin, phenindione	• Risk of excess bleeding. (➲ See Chapter 8) • Monitored by INR • Drug interaction of warfarin with antibiotics and NSAIDS
Novel oral anticoagulants (NOACs) *Action*: to prevent thrombus formation & strokes *Examples*: dabigatran, rivaroxaban and apixaban	• Risk of excess bleeding (➲ See Chapter 8) • APTT (not INR) for monitoring • Fewer drug interactions
Calcium channel blockers *Action*: reduces BP by relaxing vascular smooth muscle *Examples*: • 1. Dihydropyridines—nifedipine, amlodipine • 2. Nondihydropyridines—diltiazem, verapamil	• Gingival swelling with nifedipine

CVS = cardiovascular system; NSAIDs = non-steroidal anti-inflammatory drugs; INR = international normalized ratio; NOACs = novel oral anticoagulants; APTT = activated partial thromboplastin time

Infections and the heart

Rheumatic fever

This is an autoimmune disease triggered by a group A haemolytic strepto-coccal toxin which mimics the structure of self-antigens and results in dam-age to joints and heart valves. The illness starts in the child or young adult with a streptococcal infection—sore throat, fever, skin rash. The antibodies produced cross react with other tissues producing polyarthritis and carditis and damage continues for months up to a year while antibodies continue to circulate. Although now rare in Western Europe and North America, the disease persists in many other countries. Management is by antibiotics which may be given long term to avoid recurrence. Most commonly the damage to the heart is stenosis and calcification of aortic and mitral valves. Such lesions put the patients at subsequent risk of infective endocarditis.

Infective endocarditis (IE)

IE is a rare condition with a high mortality (around 20%). The condition arises where a bacteraemia occurs in a patient with certain types of heart defect. This can allow bacterial colonization of the heart valve surface result-ing in vegetations on the valve, loss of competency, and possible embolus.

Patients at risk of developing IE
1. Acquired valvular heart disease with stenosis or regurgitation
2. Hypertrophic cardiomyopathy
3. Previous infective endocarditis
4. Structural congenital heart disease, including surgically corrected or palliated structural conditions (excluding isolated atrial septal defect, fully repaired, ventricular septal defect, or fully repaired patent ductus arteriosus, and closure devices that are judged to be endothelialized)
5. Valve replacement

Clinical features
- Signs of systemic infection—fever, malaise, night sweats, anaemia
- New or altered heart murmur
- Petechial lesions, haematuria.

Antibiotic used to be administered prior to dental procedures which pro-voke bleeding and bacteraemia. NICE guidance has recommended that antibiotic cover is not required. This is because bacteraemia can very com-monly occur at times other than dental treatment, especially during tooth cleaning and chewing if there is inflamed gingiva. NICE also weighed the reduced likelihood of benefit from antibiotic cover against the risk of poten-tially fatal acute anaphylaxis[1].

The NICE guidance is that patients should be offered clear and consistent information about prevention, including:
- The benefits and risks of antibiotic prophylaxis, and an explanation of why antibiotic prophylaxis is no longer routinely recommended
- The importance of maintaining good oral health
- Symptoms that may indicate infective endocarditis and when to seek expert advice
- The risks of undergoing invasive procedures, including non-medical procedures such as body piercing or tattooing.

Clinical relevance

1. Patients at risk of IE are a high priority for prevention (caries and periodontal diseases). Special attention should be given to helping them achieve the best possible oral hygiene to reduce the risk of bacteraemia during toothbrushing.
2. Any oral infection that does arise must be treated promptly and effectively.
3. Patients at risk of IE may also be on anticoagulants (and so at risk of excessive bleeding) and may be a GA risk because of their heart defect.

Associations between coronary heart disease (CHD) and oral bacteria

There has been research activity investigating the role of inflammation in the development of the atheroma and a possible role of chronic infections including periodontitis. Oral bacteria have been demonstrated within atherosclerotic plaques and abdominal aortal aneurysms. The presence of pathogens—*Aggregatibacter actinomycetemcomitans* and *P. gingivalis* in periodontitis have been associated with future stroke, increased risk of myocardial infarction, and acute coronary syndrome (ACS), but no causal relationship has been proven.

Research in this area is complicated by the confounding effect of risk factors which are common to CHD and periodontal diseases, e.g. smoking, diabetes, obesity, hypertension. It is clear, however, that periodontitis is associated with the complex bacterial communities of the biofilm and host responses. Bacteraemia may occur during routine daily activities of chewing and tooth brushing and contribute to a significant cumulative exposure of the vascular system to the oral bacteria. Repeated exposure to orally derived bacteria, bacterial endotoxins, and metabolites, and systemic inflammation can directly and or indirectly induce a state of endothelial dysfunction. This may be followed by platelet aggregation, enhanced low-density lipoprotein, and cholesterol deposition in the vessel wall[2].

References

1 NICE. (2008) Prophylaxis against infective endocarditis: antimicrobial prophylaxis against infective endocarditis in adults and children undergoing interventional procedures Clinical guideline [CG64]. London; National Institute for Health & Clinical Excellence.).
2 Sanz M, D'Aiuto F, Deanfield J, Fernandez-Avilés, F. (2010) European workshop in periodontal health and cardiovascular disease—scientific evidence on the association between periodontal and cardiovascular diseases: a review of the literature. *European Heart J* 12(suppl B), B3–B12.).

Stroke (cerebrovascular accident or CVA)

Stroke is defined as a sudden onset of focal neurological deficit.
The main types of stroke are:

- Ischaemic—where the blood supply is stopped due to a blood clot (this accounts for 85% of all cases)
- Haemorrhagic—where a weakened blood vessel supplying the brain bursts, rupture of a Berry aneurysm of the Circle of Willis being the most likely cause and a subarachnoid haemorrhage results. Younger adults tend to be affected. There is a sudden onset of excruciatingly severe headache.

Risk factors include: smoking; obesity; diabetes; age; hypertension; family history; sedentary lifestyle; African or Caribbean ethnicity.

Clinical features of stroke include:

- Dysphagia
- Dysarthria (slurred speech)
- Facial paralysis
- Loss of consciousness
- Ataxia (imbalance)
- Loss of vision
- Diplopia (double vision)
- Hemiparesis (weakness on one side) or paraparesis (weakness on both sides).

Management

Fast transfer to a stroke unit will improve the outcome and the mnemonic, FAST, has been promoted to increase public awareness:

Facial paralysis
Arms weakness—arms cannot be raised
Speech problems
Time to call 999 (also protect the airway)

Careful assessment and brain imaging will be needed for diagnosis. Immediate care may include thrombolysis and anticoagulants for ischaemic stroke but management of intracerebral bleeding for a haemorrhagic stroke. Rehabilitation follows and recovery may be prolonged. Skilled assessment and multidisciplinary care is needed and a care pathway implemented to ensure coordinated care for what may be diverse impairments.

Clinical relevance

Dental treatment should be deferred if possible for 6 months following a stroke. Dysphagia will need careful assessment and may mean regurgitation into the nasopharynx or risk of aspiration. In most patients, a safe swallow is re-established within a month, probably by compensation of the unaffected side. The tongue may be weakened and drawn to one side; other orofacial muscles may not be coordinated to clear debris from the mouth and eating is likely to take longer. Extra help will be needed with oral hygiene and good plaque control may help reduce the risk from aspiration pneumonia. The dentist should liaise carefully with the physician, e.g. anticoagulants may be taken. Adrenaline should be avoided in gingival retraction and limited amounts of LA used.

Transient ischaemic attack (TIA)

TIAs comprise a sudden onset of focal CNS signs or symptoms due to a temporary occlusion of part of the cerebral circulation. They are frequently associated with partial or complete stenosis of the carotid artery system. The symptoms resolve in less than 24 hours (usually much more quickly). TIA may be followed by stroke and prophylactic aspirin is usually prescribed.

Vascular dementia

➲ See Chapter 12 for Dementia.

Pathological changes such as small vessel disease, atheroma, infarcts, and bleeds can occur throughout the brain and can contribute to cognitive impairment. Some such pathology in the brain is almost universal in people aged over 75 years. The severity, extent, and site of the lesions will determine the symptoms from mild cognitive impairment to severe dementia. In people over 80 years, there is normally a mixed picture of cognitive impairment due to vascular and neuro-degenerative (e.g. Alzheimer's disease) causes. Management of vascular dementia is based on managing vascular risk factors and comorbidities and ensuring appropriate psychosocial support to optimize quality of life.

Chapter 10

Blood

Components of blood 208
Blood cell types and functions 210
Blood cell formation (haematopoiesis) 212
Anaemia 216
Haemostasis 220
Bleeding disorders 222
Malignancy of white blood cells 226
Blood and tissue types 228

Components of blood

Blood is the transport system of the body which ensures distribution of oxygen and nutrients, removal of waste products, access to defensive systems, regulation of temperature, and the transport of hormones and signalling molecules. Whole blood is composed of fluid and cells (➲ See Table 10.1).

Table 10.1 Components of blood

Cells	Fluid (= plasma)
45% by volume	55% by volume
• White blood cells	• Mainly water
• Platelets	• Electrolytes
• Red blood cells	• Proteins—albumin, globulins, fibrinogens, and coagulation factors
	• Metabolites

Note:

Plasma refers to the fluid component of blood and is produced by centrifuging whole blood in the presence of anti-coagulant.

Serum refers to whole blood which has been centrifuged and allowed to coagulate so it lacks coagulation factors.

There are three main cell types. (➲ See Table 10.2)

- White blood cells (WBCs) or leucocytes are key parts of the body's defence system. There are six main types of white blood cell. The polymorphonuclear cells (polymorphs) have multilobed nuclei and granules prominent in their cytoplasm and so are referred to as granulocytes. The staining of these granules differentiates three types of cell: neutrophils, eosinophils, and basophils. Lymphocytes occur as T and B cells and are key to the immune system. Monocytes migrate out of the circulation and become macrophages in the tissues.
- Platelets have a key role in preventing blood loss.
- RBCs are the most numerous. They contain haemoglobin to transport oxygen and they also maintain the pH of blood.

Table 10.2 Blood cell characteristics

Blood cell type	Diameter (μ)	Count per litre of whole blood	Lifetime
Neutrophils	12–14	4–11×10^9	6 hrs
Eosinophils	12–17		4–5 hrs
Basophils	14–16		Few days or hours
Monocytes	15–20		3 days then become macrophages in liver (as Kupffer cells), lungs, spleen, lymph nodes
Lymphocytes	6–14		Few weeks or months
Platelets	1–4	140–400×10^9	10 day half life
Red blood cells	7–8	4–6.5×10^{12}	120 days

Note: The proportions are of WBCs found in circulating whole blood.
The first three cell types (neutrophils, eosinophils, and basophils) are termed granulocytes because their cytoplasm is packed with granules.

Blood cell types and functions

Neutrophils (40–70% of WBCs)

These cells are the main defence agents in blood and can attack circulating bacteria there. They are also attracted by chemotaxis to leave the circulation, squeezing out of capillaries by diapedesis to any site of inflammation. Neutrophils in turn release inflammatory mediators and phagocytose pathogens and debris, releasing a range of toxic enzymes from their cytoplasmic granules to aid destruction of phagocytosed pathogens.

Eosinophils (<1% of WBCs)

Eosinophils release inflammatory mediators and undertake phagocytosis. They take part in defence against parasites and have a role in allergy.

Basophils (<1% of WBCs)

Basophils have IgE receptors and form part of the allergic response. On activation they release histamine, heparin, serotonin & regulatory cytokines.

Mast cells

Formed in bone marrow, released into the blood as mast cell progenitors, they migrate out of capillaries into the tissue and undergo final differentiation to mature mast cells where they survive a few months. Mast cells are important in allergy and parasitic infections. When activated they release histamine, cytokines, and prostaglandins.

Monocyte–macrophage cell system

Monocytes are less than 10% of circulating WBCs and as an immature form barely participate in defence while still circulating. They migrate out into tissue, swell to form macrophages, and take the major role alongside neutrophils to combat pathogens. Macrophages main role is phagocytosis. Once activated they surround, engulf and digest pathogens and debris.

Lymphocytes (20–40% of WBCs)

There are two distinct populations of lymphocytes. B lymphocytes are responsible for humoral immunity mediated by antibodies.

The primitive lymphcytes are primed for this role by pre-processing in the liver and bone marrow. T lymphocytes are responsible for the cell mediated immunity and are primed for this role by pre-processing in the thymus. (➔ See Chapter 11)

Memory cells are derived from activated T and B lymphocytes and generated by the primary immune response to a particular antigen. They may survive for years to give a quick response to any reappearance of the antigen.

Platelets

Platelets are discoid, non-nucleated fragments only 1–2 μ in diameter. Their main function is to stop blood loss following injury by forming a platelet plug which is then stabilized by a fibrin meshwork resulting from the coagulation cascade. As part of this role they release agents that participate in the coagulation process, and other factors that attract more platelets and inflammatory cells.

Red blood cells

Mature RBCs (erythrocytes) are flexible biconcave discs of 8 μm diameter. They have no nucleus but have surface antigens which are genetically defined and which determine the blood group, mainly ABO and Rhesus.

Blood cell formation (haematopoiesis)

All the blood cells originate from stem cells in the bone marrow (myeloid tissue). In adults, the main sites are: pelvis; ribs; sternum; flat bones of the skull; proximal epiphyses of humerus and femur. The bone marrow has an enormous production capacity. It is estimated that every hour 10^{10} erythrocytes and 10^8 leukocytes are routinely produced. The process starts with a pool of haematopoietic stem cells (HSC) that are thought to be usually in a resting or non-dividing state and have the capacity to self-renew. HSCs are the source for precursors of all 10 blood cell lines: RBCs, platelets, neutrophils, eosinophils, basophils, monocytes, T and B lymphocytes, natural killer cells, and dendritic cells. There is an ordered sequence of maturation and proliferation once the stem cell is committed to a particular line. This process is finely regulated both at the level of the structured microenvironment, via cell–cell interactions and by way of the generation of specific hormones and cytokines, e.g. erythropoietin, interleukin 3, 4, and 5.

Red blood cells

RBCs develop from stem cells in the bone marrow. (➲ See Fig. 10.1)

The RBCs have a life span of about 120 days. They then become fragile and are destroyed by macrophages in the spleen and liver. Iron from RBC breakdown is recycled so that iron is reused with minimal losses.

Pluripotent stem cell

▼

Committed stem cell

▼ *Erythropoetin is released mostly from kidney (also liver) to promote and speed up RBC production in response to tissue oxygenation levels*

Proerythroblast (committed to RBC line)

▼

Erythroblast–haemoglobin is accumulating

▼

Normoblast —ejects its cell nucleus

▼

Reticulocyte

▼ *2 days maturing*

RBC (erythrocytes) released into circulation

▼ *120 days in circulation*

Fig. 10.1 Development of red blood cells.

Iron metabolism

Iron is crucial for oxygen transport (haemoglobin, myoglobin) and for electron transfer in cell respiration. Sources of dietary iron are from meat products (as haem) and nonmeat sources vegetables and cereals, as free iron. Absorption of iron is tightly controlled to avoid excess. Haem is readily absorbed by transporter mechanisms in the proximal intestines. Acid in stomach aids reduction of any ingested Fe^{3+} to Fe^{2+} which is absorbed by a transporter protein in the cell wall of enterocytes of the duodenal lining. The iron may be kept within that gut cell, bound to the storage protein apoferritin. If iron is needed elsewhere it is exported and bound to transferrin, the major plasma transport protein for iron. Most of the circulating transferrin iron comes from RBC breakdown, rather than dietary intake. Transferrin binds to receptors on developing RBC precursors in the marrow, and releases its iron for reuse. Iron is stored in skeletal muscle, hepatocytes, and reticuloendothelial system (RES). Storage is in two forms of iron–protein complexes. Ferritin is the major storage protein which binds iron within cells and a small amount of ferritin is also present in plasma. Haemosiderin is the other, less accessible, iron storage form found especially in macrophages. In the liver and spleen macrophages breakdown old RBCs and breakdown haemoglobin to globin (for amino acid pool) and haem (which is processed to bilirubin for excretion in bile).

During inflammation, iron release to the tissues is restricted, which aids in resistance to some bacterial infections. Hence iron storage as ferritin increases and there is a corresponding increase in the circulating form of ferritin in the plasma, regardless of iron status. Hence plasma ferritin levels in inflammation may mislead as to the iron status of the patient. This mechanism of sequestration of iron in inflammatory conditions appears to be the major cause of the syndrome of anaemia of chronic disease.

Platelets

Platelets develop from stem cells in the bone marrow. (➲ See Fig. 10.2).

Ageing platelets are destroyed by the macrophage system, mostly in the spleen.

Pluripotent stem cell
↓
Megakaryoctes
↓ *Thrombopoietin (from kidney and liver) stimulates production*
Fragmentation of megakyocytes
↓
Platelets
Autoregulation is by platelets destroying thrombopoietin

Fig. 10.2 Development of platelets.

White blood cells

➲ See Chapter 11, Immune System.

WBCs develop from stem cells in the bone marrow.

Production of WBCs is stimulated by:
- Colony stimulating factors (CSFs)
- Interleukins.

Pluripotent stem cell
↓

Committed stem cell differentiates into precursors of granulocytes and monocytes and precursors of lymphocytes although most lymphocytes are produced by lymphoid tissue in lymph nodes, spleen, tonsils, thymus, and Peyer's patches in the gut wall. The WBCs are stored in the bone marrow until needed. This storage normally holds a 6-day supply of such cells.

Anaemia

Anaemia is the condition of a deficiency of haemoglobin. This is defined as a haemoglobin level:
- Less than 13.5 g/100 ml for men
- Less than 12.0 g/100 ml for women.

Normally each haemoglobin molecule binds with 4 oxygen molecules, the binding of each makes the binding of the next easier. This gives a steep dissociation curve and arterial blood which is 97% saturated, 75% in the venous circulation.

The haemoglobin–oxygen dissociation curve describes the way haemoglobin's affinity for oxygen is high in the high pO_2 of the lungs but reduces as the pO_2 reduces thus releasing oxygen in the tissues. The Bohr shift describes the reducing affinity of haemoglobin for oxygen and producing increased oxygen release. This happens in response to increased temperature, CO_2 or H+ or 2,3-diphosphoglycerate (DPG). 2,3 DPG is produced in red cells and binds preferentially to the beta chain of deoxyhaemoglobin, thereby reducing the affinity of HbA for oxygen, facilitating O_2 release to tissues. 2,3-DPG causes a 'right shift' of the O_2 dissociation curve and also directly reduces the pH within the RBC which further shifts the curve to the right. Levels increase in response to high altitude, anaemia, chronic hypoxia, and chronic alkalosis.

Athletes may attempt to improve their performance by blood doping. Receiving a blood transfusion (from a donor or the athlete's own blood stored until needed) increases RBC numbers, improving the oxygen carrying capacity of the blood. It may also increase the body's capacity to buffer lactic acid. Another method is administration of erythropoietin (usually produced by kidneys, acting on the bone marrow to stimulate RBC production).

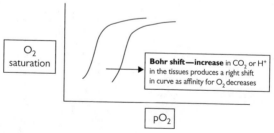

Fig. 10.3 Dissociation curve for haemoglobin.

In anaemia the oxygen carrying capacity of the blood is reduced at every pO_2. Anaemia is caused in three ways—reduced production, blood loss, or increased destruction, RBC count or haemoglobin being reduced below the normal level.

Table 10.3 Causes of anaemia

Reduced production	Drugs
	Radiation
	Infection
	Cancer
	Diet/malabsorption
	Reduced marrow stimulation
Blood loss	Obvious trauma
	Internal bleeding, e.g. ruptured ectopic pregnancy
	Chronic bleeding, , e.g from the digestive tract
Increased destruction Haemolytic anaemia	Drug interactions
	Malaria
	RBC defects
	Sickle cell disorder
	Thalassaemias

Table 10.4 Types of anaemia

Microcytic anaemia (MCV<80)	Normocytic anaemia (MCV 80–100)	Macrocytic anaemia (MCV>100)
Iron deficiency	Acute blood loss	B_{12} deficiency
Thalassaemias	Anaemia of chronic disease	Folate deficiency
	Aplastic anaemia	Alcoholism
	Haemolytic anaemia	
	Sickle cell anaemia	
MCV = Mean corpuscular volume		

Clinical relevance

Iron deficiency anaemia is the most common haematologic disorder.
Oral manifestations include
- Mucosal pallor
- Angular cheilitis
- Burning sensation
- Lingual varicosity
- Dry mouth
- Oral lichen planus
- Atrophic glossitis
- Recurrent aphthous ulcerations
- Numbness
- Dysfunction of taste
- Oral candidiasis.

Deficiency of iron, folate, B_{12}, (B_1, B_6) are often implicated in cases of oral mucosal atrophy, ulceration and risk of malignancy.

Plummer–Vinson or Paterson–Brown–Kelly syndrome (PVS)

This is a very rare condition thought to be premalignant for oesophageal or pharyngeal cancer. It is a triad of:
- Dysphagia
- Upper oesophageal web (due to formation of a postcricoid fold)
- Iron deficiency anaemia.

The pathogenesis is not fully understood but there is likely to be some genetic predisposition. The iron deficiency makes neoplastic change in mucosa more likely and reduction of iron-dependent oxidative enzymes results in gradual degradation of muscles of the pharynx allowing the postcricoid fold to form. Management is focused on correcting the iron deficiency.

Sickle cell anaemia

This is a congenital condition caused by a single base mutation in which an abnormal type of haemoglobin—sickle cell haemoglobin (haemoglobin S) is produced. Symptoms do not usually develop until around 6 months due to the persistence of foetal haemoglobin which is normal. When de-oxygenated, haemoglobin S becomes insoluble and polymerizes, resulting in RBCs ultimately losing their flexibility and becoming sickle shaped. These damaged cells have a reduced lifespan (hence haemolytic anaemia ensues). The microcirculation becomes obstructed and an infarct occurs, often pre-cipitated by cold, hypoxia, acidosis, infection, or dehydration but may occur spontaneously.

Clinical features depend on the position of the infarct but may include:
- Vaso-occlusive crises in extremities and bone causing acute pain
- Pulmonary hypertension and chronic lung disease (infection, infarction, fat embolus from necrotic bone marrow)
- Chronic problems in multiple systems.

There are degrees of severity partly depending on the genetic profile:
- Homozygous HbSS
- Heterozygous HbAS (sickle cell trait). These will not show symptoms unless subjected to extreme conditions, e.g. hypoxia during GA.
- Mixed with intermediate symptoms.

The condition is especially prevalent among patients whose origins include Africa, Middle East, India, and Southern Europe.

Clinical relevance
- Susceptible groups should be tested for sickle cell disease or trait if any general anaesthesia is planned.
- Vaso-occlusive crisis may occur in facial or dental structures and may be mistaken for a dental cause for pain.

Thalassaemias
These conditions result from genetic defects resulting in types of defective synthesis of the globin chain component of haemoglobin. There is a reduced production of either α or β globin chains. Hence erythropoiesis is impaired and there is increased haemolysis of the defective RBC. Types of thalassaemia differ in whether they are homozygous or heterozygous and in which chains are affected. There is then a range of clinical presentation from symptomless mild anaemia to severe anaemia requiring regular transfusions. There is a risk of iron overload damaging the liver, pancreas, and myocardium. The condition is distributed across Spain, Southern Europe, and the Middle and Far East.

Clinical relevance
- 'At-risk' groups should be tested for thalassaemia disease and anaemia if any general anaesthesia is planned.

Polycythaemia is the condition of increased RBC numbers commonly 6–7 million per mm³. This may occur in people living at high altitude where O_2 levels are reduced or as a response to cardiac failure where pO_2 is reduced. It also occurs in a rare genetic condition—polycythaemia vera.

Whatever the cause the circulation tends to be more viscous and slower and so the patients may appear cyanotic because of the greater degree of deoxygenation in the skin capillaries.

Drugs causing anaemia
Drugs may cause anaemia in a number of ways.
1. Drug-induced immune hemolytic anaemia
2. Drugs can cause megaloblastic anemia by impairing the cellular availability or use of folic acid or vitamin B_{12}.
3. Drugs causing blood loss (aspirin/NSAID) may cause microcytic anaemia
4. Drugs that depress bone marrow function may give rise to aplastic anaemia, e.g. chloramphenicol, phenytoin, and carbamazepine.

Summary: clinical implications of anaemia
1. Oral mucosal lesions and atrophy may be due to deficiencies of iron, B_{12} or folate.
2. Before general anaesthesia 'at risk' patients must be screened for sickle cell disorder or thalassaemias.

Haemostasis

There are three linked parts to the process of haemostasis.
- **Blood vessel constriction** occurs immediately and reduces blood loss. This is initiated by direct injury to vascular smooth muscle; reflexes initiated by local pain receptors and release of serotonin by anchored platelets and endothelial cells.
- **Platelet plug formation**—exposure of tissue factor and collagen in a traumatized blood vessel initiates the process by binding Von Willebrand's factor which binds strongly to glycoprotein receptors. Other platelet receptors bind directly to collagen. Receptor binding has two effects:
  - Tethering platelets to the blood vessel wound margins
  - Activating platelets
- This platelet plug is later supported by a tough fibrin network provided by the coagulation process.
- **Coagulation** This is a cascade which amplifies the effect initiated by factors released by damaged cells.

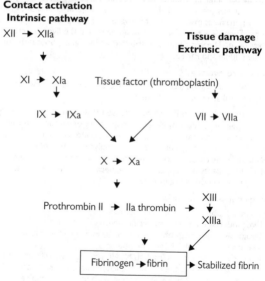

Fig. 10.4 Coagulation pathway.

Common blood tests

Activated partial thromboplastin time (APTT)

Tests the intrinsic pathway and is prolonged in heparin treatment, liver disease, haemophilia, disseminated intravascular coagulation (DIC), massive transfusion.

International Normalized Ratio (INR)

Tests the extrinsic pathway and is prolonged in warfarin treatment, liver disease, Vitamin K deficiency, DIC.

Prothrombin time (PT)

PT tests the extrinsic and common pathways. It is the time for a plasma sample to clot after a mixture of thromboplastin and calcium are added and is prolonged in warfarin treatment, liver disease, Vitamin K deficiency, DIC.

Thrombin time

It is the time taken to clot a plasma sample containing anticoagulant and excess of thrombin which have been added. This is compared with pooled normal samples. It is prolonged in heparin treatment, fibrinogen deficiency, and DIC.

Bleeding time

This test is rarely used now due to difficulties in standardization.

It is the time taken for a standardized cut to stop bleeding.

It is prolonged in platelet disorders, vessel-wall disorders, fibrinogen disorders and Von Willebrand's disease

A coagulation screen includes the following tests:

1. PT for the extrinsic pathway
2. APTT for the intrinsic pathway
3. Thrombin time or fibrinogen assay (for the final common pathway)

Note

DIC is is a complex condition of widespread activation of the clotting cascade, resulting in clots in the small blood vessels.

Bleeding disorders

The process of haemostasis is finely balanced to avoid the danger of bleeding excessively on one hand and excessive clotting and thrombus formation on the other. Of particular concern in dentistry are those conditions where excessive bleeding may occur. These conditions may be categorized into:
1. Vascular defects
2. Platelet defects
3. Coagulation disorders – inherited and acquired

Vascular defects are characterized as bruising and bleeding in mucous membranes. Possible diagnoses include the following.
- Easy bruising syndrome—commonly found in healthy females presumed due to fragility of vascular supporting tissue.
- Senile purpura, steroid purpura associated with atrophy of supporting tissue.
- Type III immune complex reaction (Henoch Schönlein purpura) following upper respiratory tract infection. Purpura develops with arthritis, haematuria, and glomerulonephritis. Usually the condition resolves spontaneously but may precipitate renal failure.
- Hereditary haemorrhagic telangiectasia—this is a rare mutation transmitted as autosomal dominant. The defect is a dilatation of the arterioles and capillaries resulting in purpura, recurrent nose bleeds (epistaxis), and chronic GI bleeding with resulting iron deficient anaemia. There may also be vascular malformations in lung, brain, and liver.
- Scurvy (vitamin C deficiency).
- Possible abuse or self -inflicted trauma should also be borne in mind as explaining bruising.

Platelet defects

Thrombocytopenia is defined as platelets $<150 \times 10^9$ litres but bleeding would not usually show clinical signs until levels were $<50 \times 10^9$ litres.
i) Abnormal platelet function commonly arises in renal disease as plasma urea and other metabolites increase, impairing platelet function. Management may include dialysis and desmopressin.
ii) Immune thrombocytopenic purpura

   In this condition platelets become coated with antibody and destroyed by macrophages. This immune response may follow a viral infection and may be associated with an autoimmune condition or chronic lymphoblastic leukaemia. Management is by steroids, IV IgG or splenectomy.
iii) Drug-induced thrombocytopenic purpura

Coagulation disorders

Von Willebrand's disease is the most common coagulation disorder and combines two defects:
- Factor VIII deficiency
- Platelet deficiency.

Von Willebrand's factor is defective here. This factor normally acts to stabilize factor VIII in plasma and to enable platelet adhesion to damaged endothelium. Investigation shows BT ↑, VIII↓. There is a range of severity. Therapy may be by administration of desmopressin in milder cases and factor VIII where bleeding is more serious.

Inherited disorders: haemophilia

Haemophilia A

Is a deficiency of Factor VIII caused by a genetic defect that is inherited as an X-linked recessive characteristic or which may occur as a spontaneous mutation. Only males develop symptoms and the prevalence is 1 in 5,000. APTT will be increased and Factor VIII reduced. There is a range of severity possible and patients will bruise easily, with bruising into joints and muscle following minor trauma. Laceration will stop bleeding because of the platelet plug and vasoconstriction but failure to form a fibrin meshwork will make the wound ooze uncontrollably after about an hour. Therapy is mostly successful with Factor VIII concentrate being regularly administered from infancy to those severely affected although inactivating antibodies may develop. Factor VIII concentrate is now treated by heat chemicals to inactivate any blood-borne viruses it contains. Patients are also routinely vaccinated against HBV. To cover any surgery Factor VIII infusion is prolonged because of the long half-life (12 hours).

Haemophilia B (Christmas disease)

Is a deficiency of factor IX and is similarly inherited as an - linked recessive, occurring in 1 in 30,000 males. This condition was famously inherited among the Romanov, Russian royal family. Therapy is by the administration of factor IX.

Liver disease

⮕ See also Chapter 5

The impairment of the liver function may impact on bleeding in several ways.

- Reduced synthesis of coagulation factors
- Functional abnormalities of fibrinogen and platelets
- Thrombocytopenia due to splenomegaly caused by portal hypertension or folic acid deficiency
- Vitamin K deficiency due to lack of bile salts in the gut (essential for absorption of fat soluble vitamins, A,D,E,K)
- DIC in acute liver failure

Vitamin K deficiency and anticoagulants

Vitamin K is essential for clotting factors II, VII, IX, X, and proteins C and S. Dietary sources include green vegetables, dairy, and soya products. It is also produced by gut bacteria. In investigation PT and APTT will be increased. Deficiency arises:

1. Haemorrhagic disease of newborn due to lack of vitamin K transfer in milk or via placenta
2. Lack of supply in severe malnutrition or due to malabsorption of vitamin K in cholestatic jaundice
3. Warfarin

Many patients seen in dental practice are taking long-term anticoagulants and these may complicate dental care. Regular monitoring of their blood levels is done by INR which is normally maintained within the range 2–4. INR of below 4 is needed to ensure safety for dental procedures which include bleeding (INR should be taken within 72 hours of the dental procedure). Obviously any attempt to reduce the warfarin dosage puts the patient at dangerous risk of thromboembolism. If the INR level is near 4 some extra bleeding is likely but it can generally be managed with local measures as above. Care is also needed over drugs which interact with warfarin—NSAIDs, amoxicillin, metronidazole, clindamycin, erythromycin.

Medications that may impair blood clotting

- Anticoagulants
  - Warfarin
  - Acenocoumarol
  - Phenindione
  - Dabigatran
  - Rivaroxaban
  - Apixaban
- Antiplatelet medication
  - Aspirin
  - Dipyridamole
  - Clopidogrel
  - Prasugrel
  - Ticagrelor
  - Abciximab/eptifibatide/tirofiban (IV preparations)
- Thrombolytic medication
  - Streptokinase
  - Alteplase
- Heparin is a short acting anticoagulant that inhibits the formation of thrombin. It is given by injection for the treatment or prevention of thrombosis or DVT after surgery. APTT is increased.

Clinical relevance

Those patients at risk of excessive bleeding need specialist advice and care for any dental treatment which carries a risk of bleeding. The following local measures may be applied in addition.

- Arrange the procedure to avoid weekends, holidays, or evenings when help may be more difficult to find
- Limit the number of teeth extracted per session
- Use a careful technique minimizing trauma
- Use LA with vasoconstrictor
- Avoid inferior alveolar nerve block injections if possible
- Gently pack the socket with absorbable dressing
- Suture the socket
- Avoid NSAIDs.

Malignancy of white blood cells

Leukaemia is a cancer of white blood cell precursors arising in the bone marrow. Leukaemia is categorized as acute or chronic.

Acute leukaemia tends to be aggressive and gives rise to immature WBC in the circulation.

- **Acute myeloid leukaemia (AML)** arises from granulocytes or monocytes. It can occur in adults or children. Prognosis for both is poor.
- **Acute lymphoblastic leukaemia (ALL)** arises from lymphocytes. It is the commonest form of leukaemia in children and has a good prognosis.

Chronic leukaemia involves proliferation of more mature cells and the prognosis is generally better than for the acute leukaemia. Adults are more commonly affected than children and the condition may be asymptomatic and found incidentally.

- Chronic myeloid leukaemia (CML)
- Chronic lymphocytic leukaemia (CLL) mostly affects people over the age of 60.

Presentation

Overgrowth of ineffective WBC leaves patients prone to infection and crowds out other blood-forming cells causing bleeding problems and anaemia. Hence signs and symptoms include:

- Recurrent infections
- Anaemia – persistent tiredness, dyspnoea, palor
- Bleeding and bruising easily
- Fever and night sweats
- Lymph node enlargement
- Abdominal swelling and discomfort
- Unintentional weight loss.

Some early signs of leukaemia may be spotted first at a dental visit.

- Lymph node enlargement
- Pale mucosa
- Poor wound healing
- Gingival enlargement and bleeding
- Mucosal bleeding (petechiae and ecchymosis)
- Recurrent infections (eg. candidiasis, herpes)
- Oral ulceration.

Treatment is by combinations of chemotherapy, radiotherapy, and bone marrow or stem cell transplantation.

Multiple myeloma is a malignancy of plasma cells.

Abnormal plasma cells take over the bone marrow and invade bone. They release only a non-functioning antibody (paraprotein). Features commonly include: bone pain in back, ribs or hips; fatigue; recurring infections; anaemia; kidney damage due to excess paraprotein; hypercalcaemia from bone resorption. Myeloma may show on radiograph as multiple punched-out radiolucencies. Treatment is by drug therapies, radiotherapy, and stem cell transplant.

Lymphoma is a cancer of lymphocytes in lymphoid tissue (not bone marrow). There are two main types.

- Hodgkin lymphoma is characterized by a particular type of abnormal cells called 'Reed–Sternberg cells'. The disease often presents as lymph node enlargement which may be in the neck.
- Non-Hodgkin lymphoma is more common in UK, usually multi-focal and has a poorer prognosis.

Treatment for the lymphomas is with combined chemotherapy and radiotherapy.

Clinical relevance

Common to all these malignancies is the potential for:

- Anaemia
- Bleeding tendency
- Impaired resistance to infection.

Regional block injections should be avoided. In addition there may be side-effects of treatments, e.g. steroids; irradiation; cytotoxic drugs; bisphosphonates. Dental care should be planned in close liaison with the patient's physician.

Blood and tissue types

Blood types

On the surface of RBCs many antigens have been identified which could give rise to antigen–antibody interactions. Among these there are two types of antigen (also called agglutinogens because of their effects) that have the most powerful impact. These are glycoproteins known as OAB and Rhesus antigens.

There are 6 types of Rhesus antigen but only type D is clinically important. Around 85% of the UK population have type D Rhesus antigen and so are Rhesus (Rh) positive. In the Rhesus system antibodies to the Rhesus antigens only usually form when there has been mixing with blood containing the different antigens. This would occur in mismatched transfusions and during development of a Rh positive foetus in a Rh negative mother. The mother develops anti-Rh antibody which diffuses across the placenta. Haemolytic disease of the newborn occurs with agglutination, haemolysis, severe anaemia, and jaundice in the newborn baby. Mothers are offered screening to detect and manage this problem.

In contrast to the Rh system, in the OAB system antibodies form spontaneously (from 2–8 months after birth, peak around 10 years and then levels decline throughout life). Antibodies develop against the agglutinogens that do not occur on the RBCs. These antibodies develop in the usual way through exposure to the antigen in food or bacteria. Blood where the RBC express type A antigen will contain anti-A antibody (agglutinogens) and cells will agglutinate/congeal if exposed to type B agglutinins. O contains both anti-A and anti-B. AB contains neither A nor B agglutinin. In transfusions the donation must be matched to the recipient's blood type, e.g. Type A blood for type A recipient.

Clinical relevance

People who have blood group O do not have A or B antigens on the surface of their RBCs. This means that they can donate blood to the other blood groups A, B, AB. However, their plasma contains anti-A and anti-B antibodies which means that they can only receive blood from another group O individual. Similarly, individuals with blood group AB can receive blood from the other three groups but cannot donate blood to them.

Donation of plasma only is the reverse of that for donation of RBCs.

Plasma from individuals with type AB blood group has no anti-A or anti-B antibodies therefore can be given to any of the other 3 groups. Those with blood group O have anti-A and anti-B antibodies in their plasma and so can receive plasma from the other blood groups, but cannot donate plasma to them.

Transfusion reactions occur when mismatched blood or plasma is administered. The RBCs of the transfused blood are attacked. Antibodies bind to the RBCs, complement is activated, proteolytic enzymes released, and RBCs rupture. A delayed reaction of phagocytosis of agglutinated cells also occurs. Both processes breakdown haemoglobin and increase levels of bilirubin which may show as jaundice. In severe cases, acute kidney failure can occur.

Table 10.5 Distribution of OAB antigens and antibodies

Blood group	Antigens on RBC surface	Antibodies in plasma	Approx. UK prevalence
O	None	Anti-a and anti-b	45%
A	A	Anti-b	40%
B	B	Anti-a	10%
AB	A and B	None	5%

Transplants and tissue types

Most body tissues also have these same antigens of the ABO type and their own set of additional antigens too. This is the basis for rejection of transplanted tissue from a donor. In addition to the ABO system, the most important antigens in graft rejection reactions are a complex known as human leukocyte antigen (HLA) and each individual has 6 such antigens from a selection of around 150 varieties. Hence there are in excess of a trillion combinations. This makes a perfect match almost impossible, except in identical twins. Fortunately some of the antigens cause minimal reaction so a perfect match is not needed. In addition, in transplantation immunosuppressive therapy is given. The target for this therapy is antibody and most especially the T cells which do most damage to donated graft tissue. Drugs include glucocorticoids, and ciclosporin. The use of these drugs puts the patient at risk of infections and also of cancers (because early cancer cells are not detected and destroyed by the immune system). Management of transplant patients thus aims to achieve an acceptable balance between the risks of graft rejection and the risks of infections and cancers.

Facial transplant

Management of extensive facial disfigurements took a leap forward in 2005 when the world's first allotransplant of a human face was performed in France. This is a type of composite tissue allotransplantation which is still experimental. The donor and recipient are matched for HLA and lifelong systemic immunosuppression is essential to control rejection. Various immunosuppressant agents have been used: corticosteroids, tacrolimus, mycophenolate mofetil, thymoglobulin, anti-IL2 receptor antibodies, X-ray irradiation. Adverse effects of immunosuppression include:

- Drug toxicity
- Opportunistic infections especially cytomegalovirus and herpes simplex infection
- Malignancies because of reduced effectiveness of immune surveillance.

Chapter 11

Immune system

Non-specific body defences *232*
Specific defences *234*
Immunization *238*
Cell-mediated response *240*
Inflammation *242*
Problems with the immune system *246*
Oral flora *250*
Dental plaque and the body's response *252*
Infection control *254*

Non-specific body defences

The body's defences comprise two systems: a non-specific (innate) and specific (acquired) defensive systems which, although independent, commonly work together. There are 2 components to the non-specific body defences:

1. Intact epithelial surfaces in places these are protected by mucous (e.g. stomach, lungs) and antimicrobial secretions (e.g. saliva, tears). Haemostasis is crucial in sealing breaches in the skin or mucosa.
2. The innate immune response (inflammation)—this is fast and non-specific.

Tissue damage (from trauma, heat, cold, radiation, or pathogens) triggers a sequence of events:

- Mast cells (these are derived from basophils which migrated out into tissue) are activated to release inflammatory mediators causing vasodilatation, increasing endothelial permeability and stimulating nociceptors.
- Macrophages and dendritic cells are activated to release inflammatory mediators, directly cytotoxic agents and cytokines (signalling molecules).
- Macrophages ingest micro-organisms, damaged cells and debris.

In addition, the complement system is activated, at first by surface molecules on the antigen and later by antibody action. The complement system is a cascade of plasma proteins which have various effects. Meanwhile damaged host cells express a PAMP-like molecule (pathogen associated molecular pattern) which attracts NK lymphocytes which destroy the cells and activate macrophages to ingest the debris. PAMP on pathogens binds to pattern recognition receptors (PRRs) on phagocytes, initiates phagocytosis, and the release of cytokines and cytotoxins.

There are a host of interacting inflammatory mediators which co-ordinate the inflammatory response (➲ See Table 11.1). Some mediators suppress inflammation, e.g. glucocorticoids, adrenocorticotrophic hormone (ACTH), products of the hypothalamic–pituitary–adrenal (HPA) axis, and some cytokines, e.g. IL-10.

Table 11.1 Inflammatory/immune response mediators

Complement—plasma proteins

A complex series of about 20 proteins with various effects:

- Inducing inflammation
- Coating antigen (opsonization) to facilitate phagocytosis
- Rupturing pathogenic cells
- Recruiting phagocytes

Cytokines—proteins/glycoproteins

Mainly synthesized by immune cells and also released from damaged cells. Cytokines help coordinate the inflammatory response by regulating differentiation and activation of immune cells.

Types of cytokine are:

- Interleukins—e.g. IL-1 produces fever, IL-8 is chemotactic, IL-4 and IL-10 decrease production of TNF
- Interferons—important against viral infection
- Chemokines—activate other cells and direct cell migration
- TNF—produces apoptosis, shock, cachexia

Histamine—an amine produced from precursor is histidine. Histamine is produced by mast cells and basophils. It is the main mediator of the immediate inflammatory response dilating arterioles and increasing vascular permeability. It is important in allergies.

Kinins—peptides

E.g. bradykinin increases vascular permeability and pain

Prostaglandins (PGs)—lipids

NSAIDs,e.g. aspirin act by preventing PG synthesis

Neuropeptides—peptides

E.g.substance P—rapidly activated vasodilator neurokinins

Nitric oxide is formed from arginine in many tissues. It has a potent vasodilator and microbicidal effect.

Platelet activating factor (PAF)—phospholipid

synthesized by many cells including PMN, monocytes, mast cells, and eosinophils. It increases vascular permeability, PMN migration, and bronchoconstriction.

Serotonin—amine released from platelets, is also a neurotransmitter. It has many inflammatory effects.

Specific defences

There are two major systems of adaptive/specific defences.
1. Humoral response mediated by B lymphocytes
2. Cell mediated response mediated by T lymphocytes (which matured in the thymus).

The two systems work very closely together. Lymphocytes are the key agents of the immune system and there are three main subgroups of lymphocytes that differentiate from precursor stem cells. These are:

B lymphocytes or B cells

B cells originating in the foetal liver from pluripotent haematopoietic stem cells mature in the bone marrow. The B cells are preprocessed with antigen receptors which will respond to a specific antigen. Together they can recognize all types of antigen (millions). From the marrow they are distributed by the circulation to lymphoid tissue throughout the body.

T lymphocytes or T cells

Just before, and for a few months after birth, stem cells originating in the bone marrow that are committed to become T lymphocytes migrate to the thymus and are each preprocessed there to react to a specific antigen (thousands). Before release from the thymus, the lymphocytes are tested against the body's own antigens and any that react are destroyed. This is the development of immune tolerance. The remainder are released into the circulation and distributed to lymphoid tissue throughout the body. In older age and with tissue damage the immune tolerance is diminished and gives rise to autoimmune disease.

Natural killer (NK) cells

NK cells are part of the innate, non-specific immune system and so need no preprocessing to prime them against a specific antigen. They contribute to defence against viral and bacterial infections and cancer. NK cells are activated by changes in surface characteristics of cells.

Major histocompatibility complex (MHC)

This is a group of about 50 genes that are important in tissue compatibility in transplants. If transplanted tissue is not closely matched to the recipient then a rapid destructive process is initiated especially by T cells which recognize MHC markers on cell surfaces. MHC class 1 is expressed on the surface of all nucleated cells and may be changed in infected or cancerous cells. T cells recognize these changes and lyse the affected host cell or secrete cytokines. Other markers for T cell activation are carbohydrate groups or antibody-mediated receptors. An important control on these cells is a strong inhibitory effect when their receptors detect normal MHC class I, thus protecting healthy cells from attack.

The role of macrophages

Macrophages originate from blood monocytes that migrate out of the circulation to patrol most body tissues and differentiate in different tissues.

- Kupffer cells in the liver
- Microglial cells in the CNS
- Alveolar macrophages in the lung alveoli
- Splenic macrophages—these are responsible to removing ageing RBC from circulation.

Macrophages lie close to the lymphocytes throughout the lymphoid tissue and play a crucial role in the immune defences. Most antigens encounter a macrophage and are phagocytosed releasing their antigen into the macrophage cytoplasm. The macrophage then presents the antigen to lymphocytes of both T and B type. This happens by direct cell-to-cell contact and results in activation of the preprocessed specific cell type for that antigen. The macrophage also secretes interleukin 1 (IL-1) which promotes growth and division of the activated cells.

Humoral response

The humoral response is the production of antibody (antigen-specific immunoglobulin) against pathogens. The response is mediated by B lymphocytes (which mature in bone marrow). The B cells have antigen receptors which can recognize all types of antigen. The antigen binds to a matching receptor on a naïve B cells which triggers clonal expansion, producing lots of B cells which transform into plasma cells and rapidly produce antibody. Some B cells transform to memory cells which persist for long periods and are the basis of immunological memory. This gives a larger number of B cells preprocessed for that specific antigen, giving a faster and more potent response at subsequent exposure to the same antigen.

If the antigen is a protein, T helper cells will join in and enhance the immune response. Non-protein antigen does not involve this mechanism.

Table 11.2 Summary of B cell types

Cell type	Function
Naïve lymphocytes	These have been preprocessed to react to a specific antigen but have not yet been exposed to that antigen for which they have been primed. They lie dormant in lymphoid tissue until this happens.
Memory cells	Long-lived cells that are produced by transformation of B cells during clonal expansion and give long term immunity responding faster and more effectively to further challenge.

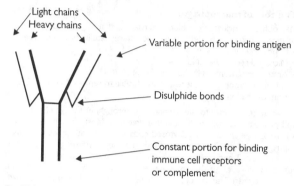

Fig. 11.1 Structure of immunoglobulin molecule.

Antibody structure
The antibody molecule is made up of four polypeptide chains, two light chains and two heavy and they are joined together by disulphide links. The Y-shaped structure has some flexibility to allow it to function better e.g. to allow more antigens to bind.
- Fc or constant portion binds with immune cell receptors or complement
- Two Fab or variable portions with hyper variability of the antigen binding section.

Types of antibody
There are 5 types of antibody which differ in their heavy chain components but share the same light chains.
- IgG is the main antibody of the secondary immune response, can cross the placenta and 80% of all serum antibodies are of the IgG type. IgG has two binding sites for antigen and can activate complement.
- IgA is found in mucous secretions (e.g. saliva, tears) and is responsible for mucosal immunity in gut and the airway neutralizing antigens before they gain entry to the body. IgA uses a dimer form in secretions (i.e. 2 antibody molecules joined). It can bind to some cells, e.g. neutrophils and some lymphocytes. It is the next most common Ig in serum after IgG.
- IgM is usually in a unit of 5 (a pentomer) each with two binding sites for antigen, so giving 10 potential binding sites. IgM strongly activates complement and is good at agglutinating organisms. IgM is the third most common serum Ig and is responsible for the primary immune response. It binds to some cells via the Fc receptors. Because of its size it does not cross the placenta.

- IgD is found on the cell surface of naïve B cell antigen receptors and may be part of the process of activation. Small amounts of IgD are found in the circulation but its role is not fully understood.
- IgE is present in low concentrations in serum but is found on the surface of mast cells and basophils, which possess an IgE Fc receptor. When bound to antigen, histamine is released, e.g. in allergy and in parasite infections.

Mechanism of action of antibodies

Antibodies have two main modes of action.

1. Direct destruction of antigen

This is usually the less potent of the two actions. Some antibodies produce lysis (cell rupture) of the pathogen. They may neutralize toxins by covering the toxic site with antibody. They may cause particles with antigen on their surface to clump together (agglutinate) and may cause soluble antigenic molecules to clump together and come out of solution (precipitate).

2. Complement activation

Complement is a complex series of about 20 proteins normally present in plasma. When the system is triggered, a cascade of reactions results in a similar way to the blood clotting cascade. The cascade may be triggered by an antigen–antibody combination which changes the configuration of the antibody molecule, uncovering a specific reactive site to which the first component of the complement sequence can bind. The cascade acts to amplify the effect and the complement system then has many potent effects.

- Opsonization by coating antigen to facilitate phagocytosis.
- Lysis (rupturing) cells.
- Chemotaxis—attracting neutrophils and macrophages.
- Agglutination—making antigen clump together for easier phagocytosis.
- Direct neutralization of some antigens.
- Activation of mast cells and basophils to release histamine and heparin and other inflammatory mediators. These will increase capillary permeability, and blood flow, inactivate or immobilize antigen.
- Other inflammatory mediators.

Immunization

The primary immune response to antigen occurs on the first occasion it is encountered. This response can take several days to get underway but part of the response is the generation of memory cells specific to that antigen. The antibody produced is mainly IgM. In a secondary response to the same antigen, memory cells are rapidly activated and mostly IgG is produced. This process is rapid, more effective and longer lasting than the primary response. This is the basis of immunization.

Protecting the population from infectious diseases can be achieved in various ways by immunization. It may be administered just to a susceptible group (e.g. as with flu vaccination) or to the whole population to achieve a herd immunity (i.e. a large proportion of the population are immune, making it difficult for disease to spread because there are so few susceptible people left to infect). The level of protection tends to fade with time and a booster may be needed in future years.

There are two approaches.

1. *Passive immunization* is achieved by giving immunoglobulin. This gives immediate but short-lived protection, e.g. against rabies.

2. *Active immunization* (also known as vaccination) is by provoking the immune system to produce a protective immune response with the use of various agents.

- Toxoid—an altered version of a toxin, e.g. tetanus
- Killed/inactivated vaccines—e.g. flu
- Live/attenuated vaccines—e.g. oral polio

Hepatitis B vaccine contains HBsAg prepared from yeast cells using recombinant DNA technology. There is also a hepatitis B immunoglobulin which provides passive immunity and can give immediate but temporary protection after accidental inoculation in a non-immune person.

Cell-mediated response

The cell-mediated response is mediated by T lymphocytes. This mechanism is crucial against intracellular pathogens, e.g. virus infections, some parasites, and mycobacteria, tumour recognition, and graft response. There are several types of T cell and they are summarized in Table 11.3.

T helper cells (also known as CD4+T cells)

The T helper cell has to have an antigen presented to it in a way it can 'recognize'. This is done by antigen presenting cells (APCs) which are macrophages, dendritic cells, and B cells. Dendritic cells are specialized to capture and process antigens, converting proteins to peptides that are presented on MHC molecules recognized by T cells. The recognition is through MHC type II (MHC class II) molecules. Once triggered the T helper cell proliferates, produces cytokines, and enhances B cell activity. In particular T helper cells produce lymphokines which:

• Stimulate proliferation and activity of cytotoxic T cells and suppressor T cells
• Stimulate B cell proliferation and activity
• Affect macrophages, stopping them migrating away and allowing them to accumulate at a site, and enhancing phagocytosis.

Some cytokines can induce class switching, i.e. changing the class of antibody produced, e.g. switch from IgG to IgM. The importance of T helper cells in defence against infections is demonstrated in HIV/AIDS, where the T helper cell activity is depleted and results in disastrous susceptibility to infection.

Cytotoxic T cells (also known as CD8+T cells)

These cells bind strongly to their matching antigen and dissolve or rupture the target cells. Examples are virus-infected cells, incompatible transplant tissue, or cancer cells.

Suppressor cells

These cells regulate and suppress the action of T helper and killer cells and may help prevent the immune system attacking the body's own tissues.

Table 11.3 Summary of types of T cell

Cell type	Function
Naïve T lymphocytes	These have been preprocessed to react to a specific antigen but have not yet been exposed to that antigen for which they have been primed. They lie dormant in lymphoid tissue until this happens.
Memory cells	Long-lived cells that are produced by transformation of T cells during clonal expansion and give long-term immunity responding faster and more effectively to further challenge.
T helper cells Also known as CD4+T cells	About 75% of all T cells Major role in controlling immune functions by releasing lymphokines.
Cytotoxic T cells Also known as CD8+T cells	These cells bind strongly to their matching antigen and dissolve or rupture the target cells. Examples are virus-infected cells, incompatible transplant tissue, or cancer cells.
Suppressor cells	These cells regulate and suppress the action of T helper and killer cells and may help prevent the immune system attacking the body's own tissues.

Inflammation

Acute inflammation

Acute inflammation is the body's initial response to cell and tissue damage. It comprises:

a) *Vascular response*
   1. Initial vasoconstriction triggered by direct stimulation of capillaries by trauma or chemicals
   2. Persistent vasodilatation
   3. Endothelial cells swell and retract

WBCs are drawn to the endothelium and adhere.

b) *Fluid exudate*—due to increased vascular permeability (due to histamine and chemical mediators from tissue damage).

c) *Cellular exudate*—cells are attracted by chemotaxis; neutrophils first, followed by monocytes. There is a sequence of margination (cells lining the walls of the capillaries) followed by migration out between endothelia.

The overall effect of this gives rise to the classic signs of inflammation locally: redness, heat, swelling, pain, loss of function.

At a systemic level, the response may include: pyrexia, malaise, rapid pulse.

Table 11.4 Mediators of inflammation and immune response

Acute inflammatory effect	Mediators
Vasodilation	Prostaglandins
	Histamine
	Nitric oxide
Increased vascular permeability	Vasoactive amines
	Bradykinin
	Leukotrienes
	PAF (platelet activating factor)
	Substance P
Chemotaxis, leukocyte recruitment and activation	C5a complement component
	Leukotrienes
	Chemokines
	IL-1 (Interleukin-1)
	TNF
	Bacterial products
Tissue damage	Neutrophil and macrophage lysosomal enzymes
	Oxygen metabolites
	Nitric oxide
Fever	IL-1 and TNF
	Prostaglandins
Pain	Prostaglandins
	Bradykinin

Chronic inflammation

Chronic inflammation results when inflammation persists and it arises when the body defences cannot resolve the problem and eliminate the cause. Examples include: autoimmune responses, prolonged infections, response to foreign bodies. The cells of this stage of inflammation are more numerous than in acute inflammation. There will be tissue destruction and repair, necrosis, and fibrosis. Macrophages are a key feature. They may accumulate as a granuloma. They may become epithelioid or coalesce into multinucleate giant cells. Plasma cells and lymphocytes are also common. Eosinophils may be a features and active against some parasitic infections. Cytokines and chemotaxins are key mediators.

Dental example of inflammation

Pupal pathology is caused most commonly by dental caries or trauma to the pulp. Trauma may arise from a physical blow to the teeth. Chemical trauma or heat may occur during dental procedures. Pulpal pain tends to be poorly localized and inflammation may be reversible, usually marked by symptoms of short intermittent pain in response to heat or cold. Pain that is prolonged after the stimulus is withdrawn or occurs spontaneously is more likely to be irreversible. Severe pain which keeps the patient awake at night is especially likely to be irreversible pulpitis or pulp necrosis. The histology does not relate closely to the symptoms.

In pulpitis, inflammation at first tends to be localized adjacent to the sources of the insult (commonly carious dentine) and there is vasodilatation and infiltrate of acute inflammatory cells. There is some destruction of connective tissue to make way for them and some odontoblasts may die. The oedema taking place within the confines of the pulp results in compression and thrombosis in the blood vessels and necrosis of the tissue.

Pulp necrosis starts coronally (possibly affecting only one root canal in a multi-rooted tooth) and proceeds towards the apex. There is chronic inflammation in the adjacent tissue and an apical periodontitis develops characterized by:

- Granulation tissue forming a fibrous wall around the lesion, proliferating endothelial cells, and immature capillaries
- Infiltration of neutrophils, macrophages, lymphocytes, and plasma cells
- Bone resorption by osteoclasts at the apex to make room for the new cells.

At this stage, the tooth gives a non-vital response to sensibility testing and may be slightly tender to pressure but may be largely symptomless. Commonly the Rests of Malassez proliferate and in some cases may develop into a cyst. In some conditions the infection may develop further, e.g. if there is a virulent organism or compromised host immunity. Consequences may include: periapical abscess, acute soft tissue infection spreading to fascial spaces, or cellulitis. See Table 11.4 for possible areas for spread.

Aftermath of inflammation

Following acute inflammation several options are possible.

- Resolution if the damage was slight
- Persistent inflammation, i.e. chronic inflammation
- Organization of exudate leading to fibrosis
- Tissue destruction leading to suppuration (pus forming).

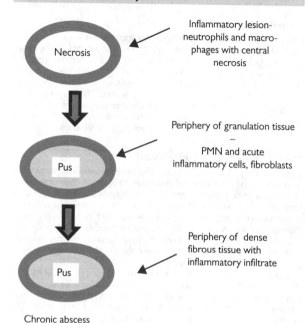

Chronic abscess

Fig. 11.2 Chronic abscess formation.

Pus occurs when macrophages and neutrophils phagocytose large numbers of bacteria and large amounts of cell debris. Most of the phagocytic cells will die, a cleft forms in the inflammatory lesion and fills with a mix of tissue fluid with:
• Dead and dying WBCs
• Dead and living organisms
• Tissue debris
• Tissue fluid and fibrin.

Pressure build up causes the abscess to expand along the path of least resistance and form an opening through the thinnest plate of bone. The sinus track to the surface is lined with granulation tissue and an excess of it may mark the entrance. If untreated dental infection may spread through soft tissue and along fascial planes as in Table 11.5.

Table 11.5 Spread of infection to tissue spaces

Teeth	Local spread	Tissue spaces
Upper incisor	Labial or palatal	
Upper canine	Labial or palatal	Canine space above muscle attachments Or nose or antrum
Upper premolar Upper molar	Labial or palatal	Buccal space above muscle attachments Or nose or antrum or pterygopalatine fossa Or peritonsillar region
Lower incisor Lower canine	Labial or lingual	Submental space Or sublingual space
Lower premolar Lower first molar	Buccal	Sublingual space
Lower second molar	Buccal	Submandibular space
Lower third molar	Buccal	Sublingual or submandibular or buccal or submasseteric or pterygomandibular or lateral pharyngeal or peritonsillar or parotid spaces

Infection spreading through connective tissue in this way is termed cellulitis. It arises in response to virulent organisms or where host defences are compromised. Spread of infection upwards towards the eye risks the potentially serious complication of cavernous sinus thrombosis with infection spreading via veins at the inner canthus of the eye to the cavernous sinus. Spread to submandibular, sublingual, submental, or pharyngeal spaces may compromise the airway and requires urgent treatment.

Problems with the immune system

Three possible problems can arise if the immune system malfunctions.
1. Reduced effectiveness of response
2. Exaggerated response – hypersensitivity
3. Response against self-antigens – autoimmune disease

1. Reduced effectiveness of response which may occur in:

Immunosuppressive therapy may be given in the treatment of:
- Autoimmune disease
- Connective tissue disease
- Transplants to suppress rejection following an organ or stem cell transplant
- Some cancers, e.g. lymphoproliferative.

Immunodeficiency diseases
- HIV and AIDS
- Congenital immunodeficiency (rare).

Chronic diseases associated with impaired immunity
- Diabetes
- Neutropenia
- Viral infections
- Cancers of blood.

Where the history reveals a potential increased susceptibility to infection the dental practitioner should liaise with medical colleagues who care for the patient to ensure a co-ordinated safe approach to management of their dental health problems.

2. Exaggerated response—hypersensitivity

Type I immediate hypersensitivity

IgE bound to mast cells and basophils responds to specific antigen by triggering release of inflammatory mediators and histamine. E.g. Anaphylactic reaction to drugs, allergies, hay fever.

Clinical application

This reaction can occur in response to foods or insect bite; in the dental surgery possible triggers are antibiotics, latex, chlorhexidine rinse. There is sudden onset and rapid progression of: facial oedema, swelling of lips/tongue, flushing and itching, chest tightness and wheeze, abdominal discomfort, rapid but weak pulse.

Management is by applying the ABCDE approach, calling for immediate help and administering 5 ml of 1:1,000 adrenaline IM and repeated after 5 minutes if no better. Adrenaline will act on:
- Alpha-receptors to reverse peripheral vasodilation and reduce oedema
- Beta-receptors to dilate the bronchial airways, increase the force of myocardial contraction, and suppress histamine and leukotriene release.

Prevention is crucial in any patients with history of allergy to dental agents and materials. A careful history taking is needed followed by referral if appropriate to a specialist centre for testing and treatment.

Type II cytotoxic hypersensitivity

IgG or IgM binds to antigen on a cell surface. Complement is activated, binds macrophages and NK cells. An example is a Rhesus negative mother who has been sensitized to Rhesus antigen during a previous pregnancy. Antibody against Rhesus factor will cross the placenta to a subsequent Rh positive foetus and cause haemolytic anaemia.

Type III complex-mediated hypersensitivity

Ag/Ab complexes are formed as result of infection or autoimmune disease. They may be localized if there is an excess of antibody or generalized if there is an excess of antigen or it is widespread through the body. Damage occurs by complement activation, platelet aggregation, degranulation of mast cells, basophils, and neutrophils. Examples of Type III hypersensitivity include glomerulonephritis and arthritis.

Type IV cell-mediated (delayed) hypersensitivity

The first exposure to the antigen primes a T cell group to respond. At later exposure to the antigen, T helper cells are activated and produce cytokines. There is a delay of around 24 hours for a localized inflammation to become obvious, macrophages are attracted and cytotoxic T cells attach to the antigen and lyse the affected cells. This reaction may occur with metals like nickel. Here the antigen is not the element itself but a complex that is formed between the metal and a body protein such as keratin.

Table 11.6 Summary of hypersensitivity reactions

Type	Response	Timescale
I Anaphylaxis E.g. Anaphylactic reaction to drugs	IgE bound to mast cells triggers release of histamine	Immediate
II Cytotoxic E.g. Rhesus incompatibility in newborn and autoimmune diseases	IgG or IgM binds to antigen and activates complement and binds macrophages and NK cells	Immediate
III Complex-mediated E.g. glomerulonephritis, arthritis	Ag/Ab complexes circulate and activate WBCs and complement which damage the target	Immediate
IV Cell-mediated Delayed hypersensitivity E.g. nickel allergy	Cytotoxic T cells attach to target cells and lymphokines are released	Delayed

3. Response against self-antigens—autoimmune disease

Although the aetiology is unknown, genetic and environmental factors contribute to susceptibility. Their effects may be highly specific to a particular organ or generalized throughout the body. (➜ See Fig. 11.3) Lichen planus has an unclear aetiology but is thought to be another autoimmune disease. Some unknown agent triggers cytotoxic CD8+ T lymphocytes to infiltrate the epithelium and damage basal cells and keratinocytes are stimulated to over-activity.

Clinical relevance

Several autoimmune diseases have manifestations in the mouth, head and neck, and the dental practitioner must be alert for these. Also treatment may involve long-term steroids or immunosuppression and again these factors must be included in management of any oral conditions.

Exaggerated response—systemic inflammatory response syndrome (SIRS)

SIRS is also named the acute phase response and is thought to be due to the systemic effects of inflammatory mediators when a large area is inflamed. The cumulative effect of this is an unbalanced state with inflammation and coagulation dominating and uncontrolled. Trauma, inflammation, or infection may trigger it. Clinically 2 or more of the following would be present:

- Fever >38°C or <36°C
- Heart rate >90 beats per minute
- Respiratory rate >20 breaths per minute or $PaCO_2$ <32 mm Hg
- WBCs high or low (>12,000/mm3 or <4,000/mm3 or >10% bands).
  Urgent treatment is required, directed at the cause and effects, in order to prevent multiple organ failure.

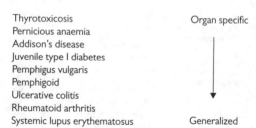

Thyrotoxicosis	Organ specific
Pernicious anaemia	
Addison's disease	
Juvenile type I diabetes	
Pemphigus vulgaris	
Pemphigoid	
Ulcerative colitis	
Rheumatoid arthritis	
Systemic lupus erythematosus	Generalized

Fig. 11.3 Effects specific to particular organs.

Oral flora

The mouth is sterile at birth but there is rapid colonization from the mother, with *Streptococcus salivarius* as an early colonizer. Several hundred species of oral bacteria are known. There is a process of chemical communication between bacteria known as quorum sensing, which enables coordinated activities and group function. This involves the production, release, detection, and group-level response to extracellular signalling molecules, called autoinducers, which in turn regulate gene expression. Collective behaviour is coordinated with benefits to defence against competitors, and adaptation to changing environments. Functions such as virulence, acid tolerance, and biofilm formation may be affected. Researchers are seeking ways to manipulate this mechanism for therapeutic benefit.

Bacteria

Also ⮀ see Dental carries in Chapter 1.

Listed below are prominent oral bacteria and conditions with which they are associated.

Gram positive cocci
- *Strep. mutans*—the most cariogenic bacteria
- *Strep. sanguinis*—an early colonizer after tooth cleaning
- *Strep. salivarius*—an early colonizer after birth
- *Strep. anginosus* group
- *Strep. sobrinus*—caries potential
- *Strep. viscosus*—caries potential
- *Strep. mitis*—caries potential

Gram-positive rods
The most numerous bacteria in plaque
- Lactobacilli—caries potential
- *Actinomyces*—caries potential and chronic suppurative disease which may start from periapical infection.

Gram-negative cocci
- *Neisseria*—an early colonizer after tooth cleaning
- *Veillonella*—strictly anaerobic with caries potential.

Gram-negative rods
- *Haemophilus*
- *Eikonella*
- *Bacteroides*

Fusobacteria—periodontal diseases

Treponema—periodontal diseases

Selenomonas—periodontal diseases

Pseudomonas—periodontal diseases

Although these genera are implicated in periodontal disease aetiology, it is thought that systemic host factors are more important.

Fungi

Candida albicans is the most common oral fungus and is a commensal found in many healthy individuals. Clinical infection can occur when conditions change:

- Change in oral flora, e.g. following antibiotic therapy
- Impaired host resistance due to drugs or disease, e.g. HIV
- Reduced salivation due to drugs, disease or irradiation
- Tissue damage due to denture movement, chemotherapy or radiotherapy.

There seem to be complex interactions between intraoral fungi and bacteria. *C. albicans* readily adheres to mucosal surfaces and *S. mutans* adheres to *C. albicans*, which may allow it to recolonize mucosal surfaces after antibiotics have reduced numbers. Associations between fungi and bacteria have also been seen to increase resistance to antimicrobials and host responses.

Viruses

A very common infection in infants is Herpes simplex. This may be subclinical or a painful gingivostomatitis. The virus then travels along the trigeminal nerve to the trigeminal ganglion where it remains lifelong and mostly dormant. Reactivation may occur in response to stress, sun, cold weather, or other virus infection, and give rise to herpes labialis lesions (cold sores). Human papilloma virus (HPV) is responsible for papillomas but is also implicated in oral cancer, especially oropharyngeal.

Dental plaque and the body's response

Also see ➔ Periodontal bone loss in chronic periodontitis in Chapter 4.

Dental plaque is a biofilm, that is, tightly packed layers of bacteria in a matrix formed of proteins from saliva and polysaccharide from bacteria. Plaque is an accumulation of large numbers and varieties of microorganisms on a tooth surface. Bacteria colonize the pellicle within minutes of brushing. Plaque has a very complex ecology with a commensal flora, competition, and antagonism between groups.

Plaque is supersaturated with calcium and phosphates but deposition of mineral crystals is inhibited by complexing agents. In the right conditions, calculus forms by mineralization of plaque with formation of crystals of hydroxyapatite as well as many other calcium phosphate salts. The rough surface of calculus is always covered in plaque. Supragingival calculus has a creamy yellow appearance and subgingival calculus tends to be brown or black, harder, and very adherent.

Gingival inflammation

Plaque biofilm releases a variety of biologically active products. These products include endotoxins, cytokines, and toxins. These molecules penetrate the gingival epithelium, stimulating gingival fluid exudate and migration of neutrophils. As the biofilm continues to proliferate, soluble compounds penetrate the sulcular epithelium. This stimulates gingival epithelium to produce chemical mediators including:

- Interleukin–1 (IL-1)
- Prostaglandins
- TNF-α
- Matrix metalloproteinases (MMPs).

These products recruit neutrophils to the area and influence chemotaxis, and can cause increased permeability of gingival vessels allowing plasma proteins into the tissue. As the inflammatory process progresses, additional mediators are produced, and more cell types are recruited to the area including neutrophils, T-cells, and monocytes. Breakdown products from the bacteria reach the circulation triggering sensitized B lymphocytes to transform to plasma cells and produce antibody specific to the antigen. Locally this will facilitate PMN phagocytosis. This combined cell-mediated and antibody-mediated response will mostly be successful in containing the attack and clinically there will be gingival inflammation.

Periodontal inflammation

In susceptible individuals the host response does not contain the threat and instead becomes destructive in the following ways.

1. Junctional epithelium proliferates and becomes increasingly permeable and ulcerated;
2. More bacterial products flood in;
3. More macrophages, lymphocytes are attracted to the area and many PMNs infiltrate the tissues;
4. PMNs secrete destructive enzymes and inflammatory mediators including MMPs, enzymes that degrade extracellular matrix and basement membrane and which break down the gingival and periodontal fibres;

5. Prostaglandins, interleukins, and TNF stimulate local osteoclasts to resorb alveolar bone;
6. As the junctional epithelium is destroyed it regrows at a more apical position and a pocket is formed;
7. As the biofilm migrates apically along the root surface conditions allow more anaerobic and gram-negative species to proliferate.

Periodontitis and systemic disease

There has been a lot of research into possible links between periodontal disease and a number of systematic conditions: cardiovascular disease; cerebrovascular diseases; diabetes; respiratory diseases; mental disorders (e.g. depression); obesity; rheumatoid arthritis; osteoporosis; and complications of pregnancy. For some of these a possible bidirectional relationship is suggested between periodontitis and systemic disease. This is especially well seen in type 1 diabetes. Periodontitis is associated with increased susceptibility to diabetes and poor glycaemic control worsens the periodontal condition.

The search for causal pathways has focused on lipopolysaccharide in the cell wall of Gram-negative bacteria, which stimulates host cells to produce a number of inflammatory mediators (e.g. prostaglandins and nitric oxide) and potent proinflammatory cytokines (e.g. TNF-α, IL-1, IL-6). Such inflammatory mediators and bacterial products finding their way into the blood stream and to distant organs may, in susceptible hosts, be key to initiating other conditions.

Infection control

Instrument decontamination

Current guidance must be followed to ensure safe processing of used instruments. HTM-01-05 outlines the following steps.

1. Cleaning with washer disinfector or ultrasonic cleaner (manual cleaning carries a high risk or sharps injury)
2. Inspection (and recleaning if needed) to ensure all blood and debris is removed
3. Sterilization with pressurized steam (typically 134–137°C for 4 minutes)

There are two types of sterilizer. One operates by passive displacement by steam; the second type is vacuum forming and gives better penetration of steam especially for use with hollow instruments like handpieces and it allows loads to be packaged prior to sterilization. The subsequent processes of wrapping, storage, and transportation must be carefully done to ensure no contamination occurs. There are some areas of especial difficulty in achieving total eradication of risk from the decontamination process. Sterility is unlikely to be achieved in the lumen of handpieces because of the presence of lubricant. Prions (the abnormal proteins associated with vCJD) are especially resistant to decontamination processes.

Variant Creutzfeldt-Jakob Disease (vCJD)

This is a neurodegenerative condition. The causative agent is a prion (self-replicating misfolded protein). First diagnosed in 1994, 2 years later the link was made between vCJD and bovine spongiform encephalitis (BSE), a neuro-degenerative disease of cattle. Initial cases were contracted from meat contaminated with prions and measures were put in place preventing meat from infected cattle from entering the food chain. But once humans are infected no symptoms may be evident for decades. Hence the prevalence in the UK of people carrying vCJD is uncertain with estimates ranging widely from 1:2,000 to 1:20,000 and incidence of 1 new case in a million per year worldwide.

Risk of transmission of vCJD

Blood, blood products, and organ transplants present a potential risk of transmission so, from 1999, the UK no longer sourced plasma from its inhabitants, and instituted leukocyte depletion (removal of WBCs) from blood transfusions. Animal studies have shown dental instruments to be a potential risk of transmission for vCJD. Although no such cases of transmission in the dental clinic have been recorded they may have gone undetected. Prions are especially found in nervous tissue and resist normal decontamination, with cleaning of organic debris being especially crucial. Hence endodontic instruments are now for single use (or for reuse only on the same patient).

Table 11.7 Fate of airborne particles

Particle size	Penetration	Timescale
50–100 μm splatter	Deposit on any surface within 1 m	Deposit within minutes
10–50 μm aerosol	Pharynx	Remain airborne for hours
<10 μm aerosol	Lung to secondary bronchioles	Remain airborne for days
<2.5 μm aerosol	Terminal bronchioles/alveoli	Remain airborne potentially for weeks

Splatter and aerosol represent a major source of risk around the dental surgery as illustrated in Table 11.7.

Harm reduction is by:
- Use of protective glasses
- Use of mask by operator and assistant
- Pretreatment mouth rinse
- Use of high volume aspirator
- Well-ventilated surgery
- Use of rubber dam
- Use of zoning and protective covers to surfaces.

Dental unit water lines

Dental units contain metres of plastic tubing with a 1–2 mm lumen. Gram-negative aerobic bacteria, fungi, and amoebae may be found in the biofilm that forms on the inside of these tubes. Mostly these are harmless except in medically compromised patients, but there may also be *Pseudomonas*, *Legionella*, and non-tuberculosis *Mycobacterium* species. It is crucial to follow the manufacturer's instructions and current guidelines in the care of the dental unit water lines e.g:
- Disinfection systems on the water line
- Anti-retraction valve on handpieces (to prevent oral fluids being drawn into the tubing and add to the flora)
- Handpieces should be operated to discharge water and air for 20–30 s between patients and for 2 minutes at the start of the day
- Periodic testing of the output water.

Protection of staff

All staff must use personal protective equipment (PPE) appropriate to the tasks they are performing. At the chairside this will usually comprise: gloves; face mask; eye protection; apron or tunic. A visor may give added protection against splatter. Chairside staff should have their arms bare below the elbows or use disposable plastic sleeve covers. Gloves must be changed after each patient or if puncture/contamination occurs. Heavy duty rubber gloves should be used for some manual cleaning tasks. Face masks lose their effectiveness with time and if they become damp. Blood spillages must be tackled immediately. Protective clothing must be used for this and 10,000 ppm hypochlorite solution applied for at least 5 minutes.

Inoculation injuries are incidents where a contaminated object or substance breaches the integrity of the skin or mucous membranes or comes into contact with the eyes. Precautions against such injuries include: PPE must be used; needles must not be recapped after use or an appropriate device must be used to control the risk of injury. Burs and tips of sonic/ultrasonic scalers should be removed from handpieces after use. After a sharps injury any wound should be encouraged to bleed and then washed thoroughly with soap and running water. Then a risk assessment should be done for transmission of infection. Occupational health advice should be sought. If there is a significant risk for transmission of HIV then post-exposure prophylaxis (PEP) should be started. This is a 4-week course of anti-retroviral drugs. Approximate risks for a non-immunized person contracting disease after an inoculation injury from an infected patient are stated as: 30% for hepatitis B; 3% for hepatitis C and 0.3% for HIV. All staff who undertake exposure prone procedures should have appropriate immunizations. Crucial among these is immunization against hepatitis B. (➲ See Chapter 5)

Central nervous system

Nerve conduction 258
Facial and dental pain 260
How do we appreciate pain? 262
The anatomy of facial skin sensation 264
The cranial nerves 266
The autonomic nervous system 268
Modifying patient behaviour 274
Local anaesthesia 276
Providing dental local anaesthesia 278
Sedation, general anaesthesia, and analgesia 280
Drug problems in dental practice 282
Dementia 284

Nerve conduction

Nerve impulses are conducted to the CNS in axons.
- With a mild (subthreshold) stimulus, no electrical activity is recorded in the nerve.
- Increasing the stimulus strength (to a suprathreshold level) causes an action potential, which is a rapid depolarization of the nerve.
  - During and immediately following the action potential, the nerve membrane becomes unresponsive to further stimulation (a refractory period).
  - This ensures that the action potential only propagates in one direction, i.e. the action potential does not depolarize the membrane where the action potential has just been.
- Increasing the stimulus strength still further does not produce a greater action potential than a suprathreshold response.

If successively larger stimuli are now applied to a whole nerve, increased electrical activity can be recorded. This is not due to increased response of the individual axon but to the activation of other nerves with a higher threshold.

Origin of the resting potential

- There is a resting potential of about -70mV across the nerve membrane. This arises from potassium ions diffusing out of the cell due to their greater concentration within the nerve. Negatively charged ions are unable to follow due to selective permeability of the membrane. Further outward diffusion of potassium ions is prevented by the potassium ion voltage gradient.
- The higher sodium ion concentration outside the cell tends to increase the membrane potential as these ions have a tendency to move into the cell. The membrane permeability to sodium ions is considerably less than for potassium ions, so the influence of the influx of the sodium ions on the resting membrane potential is much less.

Origin of the action potential

- A depolarization of the nerve membrane causes an increase in the ionic permeability to sodium ions. Sodium ions move into the nerve causing the membrane potential to become positive.
- The membrane permeability for sodium ions decreases rapidly and is followed by an increase in the potassium ion permeability which returns the membrane potential back to normal.
- The flow of action potential current depolarizes the adjacent nerve membrane, generating an action potential in that region. In myelinated nerves, generation of the action potential is limited to those regular regions along the nerve where the myelin is absent. This means that the conduction velocity is much greater in myelinated than in unmyelinated nerves.
- The equilibrium potential is maintained over the long-term by a sodium-potassium ion ATPase which actively transports sodium ions out of the cell and potassium ions into the cell. As this is against the concentration gradient for these ions, energy is consumed.

Clinical relevance: nerve action potential is 'all or none'

Depolarization below a threshold does not elicit an action potential. It requires a depolarization of a particular magnitude for the action potential to be generated. Action potentials are generated by the flow of ions and as they do not require energy at the point of their generation, they are therefore of constant magnitude along the length of the nerve.

The velocity of conduction in a nerve is determined by its diameter and whether the nerve is myelinated or not.

Synaptic transmission

- There is no cellular continuity between nerves.
- When the action potential reached the terminal end of the pre-synaptic nerve, it stimulates the release of a neurotransmitter into the synaptic gap between the two nerves.
- The neurotransmitter diffuses across the gap and binds with a receptor on the post-synaptic membrane.
- This causes either a more negative post-synaptic nerve potential (inhibitory post-synaptic potential) or a depolarization (excitatory postsynaptic potential).
- The neurotransmitter is released from the receptor and is then enzymatically degraded or is reabsorbed by the nerves.

A number of substances are known to act as neurotransmitters in the CNS. Some drugs modify nervous transmission by either blocking the receptors or inhibiting the enzymes which degrade them.

- Depression is often treated with drugs that inhibit the enzymatic breakdown of catecholamine.
- In Parkinson's disease, there is loss of dopaminergic neurons in the substantia nigra. Symptoms include slow movement, rigidity and a resting tremor. It is treated with levodopa and dopamine agonists.

Facial and dental pain

What are the anatomical pathways for pain?

From the teeth and face?

The trigeminal nerve provides sensation to the face, teeth and nasal cavity. When pulpal tissues are stimulated, only the sensation of pain is appreciated. The nerve fibres terminate in both the sensory nucleus and the spinal nucleus of the trigeminal ganglion, where secondary neurones relay to the thalamus. Tertiary neurones further relay the painful stimulus to the cerebral hemisphere and hypothalamus.

From the periphery?

Nociceptive fibres relay with second order neurons in the dorsal horn of the spinal cord in an ordered manner, with processing much influenced by descending axonal activity from the brainstem. The nociceptive input is relayed to the lateral thalamus, limbic system, and somatosensory cortex.

Central processing of painful stimuli

Pain-specific neurons synapse in the substantia gelatinosa of the spinal cord, and the second interneuron crosses the midline and relays in the thalamus or lenticular formation.

- There is an increased response from the spinal cord interneurons following repeated afferent painful stimuli (called 'central sensitization'). This results in a heightened painful response to mild innocuous stimuli. This is an example of central neuronal plasticity.
- The area of skin adjacent to an injury exhibits an exaggerated pain sensation following mild stimulation (called 'peripheral sensitization'). Stimulation from nociceptive nerve fibres over the area of injury causes the release of histamine and 5-hydroxytryptamine in the adjacent uninjured skin. This cause further excitation of nociceptors.
- There is a descending neural pathway from the cortex and hypothalamus that inhibits the afferent pain pathway. The descending pathway passes through the midbrain and medulla and synapses with the spinal cord interneurons (or nucleus caudalis of the trigeminal nerve).

Why is dentine painful when dried with air?

The 'hydrodynamic hypothesis' suggests that fluid movement in dentinal tubules stimulates the small Aδ nerve fibres. However, dental afferent nerves mainly consist of larger Aβ-fibres, but may function as low threshold mechano-sensitive fibres involved in the neural processing of noxious stimuli. Cold stimuli cause dentinal fluid to flow out from the pulp, while warm stimuli cause fluid to move into the pulpal tissues. The nerve fibre receptor which detects the fluid movement has not been found, but a possible candidate which has been found in dental afferent fibres and may act as a mechanical transducer is TRPV1 (transient receptor potential vanilloid receptor subtype 1). This receptor is also activated by heat. Nerves are not found further peripherally than the inner dentine and mostly terminate in the odontoblast and predentine layers.

Neonatal rat and human odontoblasts also possess TRPV1. The presence of odontoblast membrane mechanoreceptors and an ability to generate action potentials in vitro is evidence that they may act as sensory transducers. Odontoblasts do not contain neurotransmitter vesicles and do not form synapses with nerves, therefore the mechanism of how odontoblasts stimulate adjacent sensory neurones is not known. The most recent evidence suggests that adenosine triphosphate (ATP) may be released from the odontoblast and stimulate purinergic receptors on the adjacent nerves.

Innervation of the teeth

The nerves entering the tooth consist of Aδ, Aβ, and unmyelinated C fibres. The nerves branch extensively.

- Plexus of Raschkow is a branching network of nerve fibres that is present below the odontoblast layer of cells.
- Some nerve fibres enter the coronal dentinal tubules.

Clinical relevance

Dentine hypersensitivity is common. Patients often report a sharp painful response to dentine stimulation followed by a longer lasting ache. The sharp response is due to the stimulation of Aβ and Aδ nerve fibres. The aching component may be due to stimulation of unmyelinated C fibres, whose response is dramatically increased by inflammatory mediators. There are three hypotheses explaining dentine sensitivity:

- Local anaesthetics do not eliminate pain when applied to exposed dentine. This would indicate that nerves in the dentine are not the primary mechanism for dentine sensitivity.
- Odontoblasts may be sensory receptors
- Receptors in the pulp may respond to fluid movement in the dentinal tubules.

Neurotransmitters and pain perception

Substance P

- Dentine-bonding agents can cause the release of substance P in the dental pulp.
- Substance P activates vasodilation and inflammation when released from the peripheral endings of sensory nerves.
- Substance P is an important neurotransmitter involved in stress and in addiction-related behaviours.

Endorphins

- Cause pain relief
- Inhibit the release of the inhibitory neurotransmitter gamma-aminobutyric acid (GABA)
- Exogenous opiod drugs compete at the receptors with endogenous endorphins.

How do we appreciate pain?

Pain is more than the transmission and reception of nerve impulses in the brain cortex. The experience of pain also involves the affective or emotional reaction to pain and is intimately involved with its experience. It may be a major factor influencing the pain experienced by an anxious patient undergoing discomfort when treated by their dentist.

Pain can be caused by the reaction to inflammation of tissues following trauma or to damage to nerves. Previous pain episodes can cause the patient to develop chronic pain (i.e. lasting over 3 months). It is now thought that patients develop a chronic pain condition as a result of increased sensitivity of the CNS following nociceptive input from repeated tissue damage. Experimental results in animals have shown that these changes are permanent and involve changes in neural pathways and synapses. This may explain the limited success rate in treating chronic pain.

Following tissue damage, local inflammation is induced by the release of bradykinin, substance P, serotonin, and prostaglandins, which cause a sensation of heightened pain (or hyperalgesia).

The processing and modification of the nociceptive impulses is carried out by

- The amygdala (involved in the autonomic response to pain)
- Hypothalamus and thalamus (involved in inhibiting the ascending nerve impulses at the midbrain)
- Insula (involved in empathy) and anterior cingulate cortex (assesses the relevance to motivational effort).
- Midbrain and hippocampus.

In experiments on patients with constant post-surgical pain, these areas received a greater blood flow.

Abnormal sensation

Dysaesthesia
- An abnormal, painful touch sensation.

Paraesthesia
- A tingling sensation. Causes include shingles, diabetes, multiple sclerosis, and carpal tunnel syndrome.

Allodynia
- Mild stimuli are felt as being painful.

Clinical relevance
The commonest cause of altered sensation is due to trauma to either the inferior alveolar or lingual nerves. Lingual nerve damage affects taste sensation. This can occur during removal of third molar teeth, endodontics, or implant surgery. The lingual nerve may be damaged during inferior alveolar block injections.

Risk factors for extraction of an impacted third molar (indicating a close proximity of the tooth to the inferior alveolar nerve) include:

- Displacement of the inferior alveolar nerve canal on radiograph.
- An increased radiolucency of the tooth roots on radiograph.
  A radiolucent band may be seen across the apex of the impinging tooth.
- There may be an interruption to the corticated lamina dura of the inferior alveolar nerve. On radiographs, the corticated margins normally appear as white 'tramlines' but these can seem narrowed or constricted at points over the impinging root.
- Deviation of the impinging tooth root or a sudden change in the direction of the tramlines.

Trigeminal neuralgia

The characteristic presentation is of severe electric shock type pain elicited by gently touching specific trigger points on the skin.

Multiple sclerosis (MS) as an example of a relatively common demyelinating condition that many dentists will come across in practice. Trigeminal neuralgia can be a clinical manifestation of MS. The majority of cases of trigeminal neuralgia are caused by pressure on the nerve, usually from an artery or vein. Demyelination and spontaneous generation of impulses in the nerve may result. This causes severe, paroxysmal pain usually lasting up to a few minutes at most. On examination, there are no changes in sensation, so diagnosis is highly dependent on obtaining a detailed clinical history. Carbamazepine is the drug treatment of choice.

Migraine

Migraine is manifested by a headache with visual disturbances and sensitivity to smells and sound, and is often accompanied by nausea and vomiting.

Migraine is accompanied by sensitization of perivascular pain receptors. Other factors in the aetiology include hyper-excitability of cortical neurons and an altered processing of pain. Chronic migraine is associated with persistent cortical hyper-excitability and cutaneous allodynia.

Burning mouth syndrome

Burning mouth syndrome is characterized by a burning sensation in the mouth with no obvious cause being visible. A majority also complain of taste disturbances or dry mouth. It has been proposed that the pain in this condition is related to an increased number of fungiform papillae and pain fibres in the mouth, combined with additional loss of central control of pain inhibition.

The anatomy of facial skin sensation

The trigeminal nerve
The trigeminal nerve innervates the facial skin, providing sensory input to the CNS. It has three main divisions:
- Ophthalmic division supplies:
  - The skin of the forehead and scalp
  - Skin of the nose
  - Conjunctiva and skin over the upper eyelid
- Maxillary division supplies:
  - Skin over the lower eyelid, side of the nose and the cheek
  - Gingiva from the midline to the second premolar region
  - Skin covering the zygomatic bone
- Mandibular division supplies:
  - The external acoustic meatus, tympanic membrane, and some of the skin of the ear and temple (via the auriculo-temporal nerve)
  - Skin over the cheek, buccal gingivae of the second and third molar teeth (via the buccal nerve)
  - Skin of the lower lip and the anterior labial gingiva (via the mental nerve).

The great auricular nerve (a branch of the cervical plexus) supplies skin over the ear, parotid gland and angle of the mandible.

The mandibular division of the trigeminal nerve
The inferior alveolar nerve passes medial to the lower head of the lateral pterygoid muscle and passes between the medial pterygoid and the ramus of the mandible. The inferior alveolar nerve enters the mandibular canal of the mandible at the mandibular foramen. The inferior alveolar nerve takes a course that either lies just below the apices of the teeth or runs close to the lower border of the mandible. It supplies sensory innervation to the molar and premolar teeth.

At the mental foramen, the inferior alveolar nerve divides into:
- Incisive nerve (which supplies the sensory innervation to the canine and incisor teeth and labial gingiva)
- And the mental nerve (which innervates the skin over the lower lip and chin).

The gingivae buccal to the molar teeth are supplied with sensory sensation by the buccal nerve (also called the long buccal nerve). This nerve takes its origin from the anterior trunk of the mandibular nerve. The other branches of this trunk (masseteric nerve, deep temporal nerve and nerve to the lateral pterygoid) have a motor function.

The maxillary division of the trigeminal nerve
The maxillary nerve divides into:
- A meningeal branch in the cranial cavity
- Ganglionic, zygomatic and posterior superior alveolar nerve branches in the pterygopalatine fossa.

Ganglionic branch
These nerves pass through the pterygopalatine ganglion to supply sensory innervation to the mucosa of the soft palate, nasopharynx, palate, and lateral wall of the nose.

The zygomatic branch
This nerve carries secretomotor parasympathetic fibres to the lachrymal gland. The zygomatic nerve divides into zygomaticofacial and zygomatcotemporal branches.

Posterior superior alveolar nerve
The posterior superior alveolar nerve supplies the sensory innervation to the maxillary sinus, maxillary molar teeth, adjacent buccal gingiva and cheek.

The middle superior alveolar nerve and the anterior superior alveolar nerve leave the infraorbital nerve in the infraorbital canal.

Middle superior alveolar nerve
The middle superior alveolar nerve has a variable course but, if present, innervates the premolar teeth.

Anterior superior alveolar nerve
The anterior superior alveolar nerve innervates the incisors and canine teeth. It also contributes to the sensory innervation of the mucous membrane at the lateral nasal wall, floor of the nose, and nasal septum.

All three superior alveolar nerve branches (anterior, middle, and posterior) form part of the superior dental plexus.

The infraorbital nerve has the following cutaneous branches:
• Palpebral branches supplying the lower eyelid and cheek
• Nasal branches supplying the skin of the nose
• Superior labial branches innervating the upper lip and labial gingiva.

Referred pain

Referred pain is felt in a region different from where the painful stimulus is present. There is extensive convergence of sensory input from the facial region onto the subnucleus caudalis. The convergence of stimuli may prevent the CNS from interpreting the source of the pain. Alternatively, repeated stimulation may cause sensitization of brainstem neurons making them more responsive and increasing their receptive area. The latter theory may explain the delayed onset for referred pain as time is needed for the necessary sensitization to take place.

The cranial nerves

⮕ See Table 12.1 for the cranial nerves and their functions.

Clinical relevance

Neck dissection

Radical neck dissection to remove squamous cell carcinoma removes the sternocleidomastoid muscle, internal jugular vein, and accessory nerve. This causes considerable postoperative morbidity. Selective neck dissection avoids the unnecessary mutilation and is used primarily for removal of occult metastasis or in patients who are at risk of metastatic spread to the cervical lymph nodes.

Table 12.1. Summary of the cranial nerves and their function

Cranial nerve	Function
Olfactory nerve (I)	Smell
Optic nerve (II)	Vision
Oculomotor nerve (III)	Contraction and dilation of the pupil. Movement and proprioception of eye muscles (except superior oblique and lateral rectus muscles)
Trochlear nerve (IV)	Movement and proprioception of the superior oblique eye muscle
Trigeminal nerve (V)	Sensation of the facial skin and mucous membranes of the head and neck. Motor supply to the muscles of mastication
Abducent nerve (VI)	Movement of the lateral rectus muscle of the eye
Facial nerve (VII)	Movement of the muscles of facial expression. Taste to the anterior two-thirds of the tongue. Afferent sensation to the external auditory meatus, soft palate, and pharynx. Secretomotor to the submandibular, sublingual, and lacrimal glands.
Vestibulocochlear nerve (VIII)	Balance. Hearing
Glossopharyngeal nerve (IX)	Taste sensation to the posterior third of the tongue. Secretomotor to the parotid gland. Motor sensation to the stylopharyngeus muscle. Afferent sensation to the mucous membrane of the tonsil, pharynx, soft palate
Vagus nerve (X)	Regulates heart rate, gut movements and sensation, coughing, skin sensation in the posterior wall of the external auditory meatus
Accessory nerve (XI)	Efferent supply to the muscles of the pharynx (eg levator palati muscle), larynx, sternocleidomastoid, trapezius.
Hypoglossal nerve (XII)	Efferent supply to extrinsic and intrinsic tongue muscles (except palatoglossus)

Consequences of lesions of nerves controlling eye movement
The oculomotor nerve (III), trochlear nerve (IV), and abducens nerve (VI)
are responsible for eye movement.
➲ See Table 12.2 for functional disturbance of paralysed nerves.

Table 12.2. Functional loss following paralysis of nerves causing eye movement

Nerve paralysed	Functional disturbance
Oculomotor n	Ipsilateral eye affected: drooping of the eyelid (ptosis)
	Dilation of the pupil which does not respond to light. Loss of focus for near objects as the shape of the lens cannot be changed.
	The lateral rectus and superior oblique muscles are unaffected and so cause the eye to be rotated inferiorly and laterally.
Trochlear n	Vertical diplopia. The ipsilateral eye is pulled upwards by the unopposed action of the other eye muscles.
Abducent n	This nerve innervates the lateral rectus muscle, which moves the eye laterally. Abducent nerve paralysis causes the eye to deviate medially (called esotropia).

The autonomic nervous system

The autonomic nervous system is composed of the sympathetic and parasympathetic systems. The autonomic nervous system controls smooth muscles, glandular secretion, and functions of the cardiovascular system. Both sympathetic and parasympathetic efferent systems have nicotinic acetylcholine receptors at their ganglia (⮕ See Fig. 12.1).

- The parasympathetic system has muscarinic acetylcholine receptors at the effector organ.
- The sympathetic system has mainly noradrenergic receptors at its effector organs (the exceptions are the eccrine sweat glands and the adrenal medulla which have acetylcholine receptors).
- The sympathetic and parasympathetic systems tend to work in opposition to one another.

Drugs which act on the ganglionic nicotinic acid acetylcholine receptors have such widespread effects that they have limited usefulness. Similarly, there are no applications in routine dental practice for adrenergic antagonists. The type of adrenergic receptor in an organ ($\alpha 1$, $\alpha 2$, $\beta 1$, and $\beta 2$ will determine its response to the selective adrenergic agonist and antagonistic drugs.

- $\alpha 1$ receptor stimulation results in constriction of blood vessels.
- $\alpha 2$ receptors are present on the presynapse. When stimulated by the synaptic release of norepinephrine (also called noradrenaline) these receptors prevent further release in a feedback mechanism.
- $\beta 1$ receptor stimulation causes an increased heart rate.
- $\beta 2$ receptor stimulation causes dilation of blood vessels in the muscles and bronchodilation.

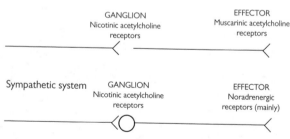

Parasympathetic system

GANGLION
Nicotinic acetylcholine
receptors

EFFECTOR
Muscarinic acetylcholine
receptors

Sympathetic system   GANGLION
Nicotinic acetylcholine
receptors

EFFECTOR
Noradrenergic
receptors (mainly)

Fig. 12.1 The autonomic nervous system: ganglion and effector receptors.

Pharmacology of the autonomic nervous system

Anticholinergic drugs

There are many cholinergic synapses in the CNS with a mainly excitatory effect. Some drugs used to treat psychosis and schizophrenia, such as haloperidol and chlorpromazine, have an anticholinergic action.

Other examples of anticholinergic drugs are

- Those with an antihistamine action (such as diphenhydramine)
- Tricyclic antidepressants (such as imipramine or amitriptyline).

Adrenergic neurotransmitters

The action of adrenergic neurotransmitters at the synapse is mainly by neuronal re-uptake. This action is inhibited by tricyclic antidepressants.

Biotransformation of epinephrine (adrenaline) in local anaesthetic

Adrenergic drugs, such as epinephrine and corbadrine, are used in local anaesthetics. They are both metabolized in the liver, mainly by catechol-O-methyltransferase (COMT). MAO inhibitors do not prevent the metabolism of epinephrine administered in local anaesthetics.

Epinephrine is used in local anaesthetics to provide vasoconstriction of submucosal blood vessels and delay the absorption of the local anesthetic.

Anatomy of the autonomic nervous system in the head and neck region

The cranial parasympathetic effector fibres leave the brainstem in cranial nerves III, VII, IX, and X and synapse in the ganglia. Postganglionic fibres then supply the sphincter pupillae, ciliary muscles, lacrimal glands, and salivary glands in the head and neck region (➔ See Table 12.3). The sympathetic fibres, with their pre-ganglionic cell bodies in the intermediolateral cell column of the spinal cord, leave the thoracic and lumbar spinal cord, synapse in the ganglia and usually have long post synaptic fibres to the effector organ.

The autonomic nervous system has a sensory component with cells located in the dorsal root ganglion. These cell bodies have peripheral and central projections to the spinal cord. The central projections form reflexes with the autonomic preganglionic neurons or interneurons or project to higher centres in the CNS. In the spinal cord, nerves from the somatic and autonomic systems are integrated and project to the same neuron. This allows integration of information and explains how damage to the viscera can be appreciated as pain from the nearby skin (called referred pain). One example is the pain from angina which is often perceived as acute retrosternal pain.

The ganglia in the head and neck region (Table 12.1) have sympathetic, parasympathetic, and somatic sensory afferent nerves passing through, but only the parasympathetic fibres synapse in the ganglion.

Table 12.3 Autonomic nervous system in the head and neck

Cranial nerve	Preganglionic nerve	Ganglion	Effector organ
Oculomotor nerve	Oculomotor nerve	Ciliary ganglion	Sphincter pupillae and ciliary muscles
Facial nerve	Greater petrosal nerve	Pterygopalatine ganglion	Lachrymal gland
Facial nerve	Mandibular division of trigeminal nerve	Submandibular ganglion	Submandibular and sublingual salivary glands
Glossopharyngeal nerve	Lesser petrosal nerve	Otic ganglion	Parotid salivary gland

Lachrymation

The parasympathetic root of the facial nerve leaves the pons and enters the pterygopalatine ganglion via the nerve of the pterygoid canal. There the nerve fibres synapse and postsynaptic fibres join the zygomatic branch of the maxillary nerve. The secremotor fibres travel in the zygomatic nerve and lachrymal nerve to the lachrymal gland. The lachrymal nerve is a branch of the ophthalmic nerve.

Sympathetic nerve fibres leave the carotid plexus and form the deep petrosal nerve. These fibres join the nerve of the pterygoid canal and pass through the pterygopalatine ganglion without synapsing. The branches of the pterygopalatine ganglion to the nose, orbit, and palate contain sympathetic fibres.

Salivation

Fibres from the superior salivatory nucleus in the pons enter the facial nerve and leave via the chorda tympani nerve. This unites with the lingual nerve (a branch of the mandibular division of the trigeminal nerve) and supplies secretomotor fibres to the sublingual and submandibular salivary glands. Taste sensation to the anterior two-thirds of the tongue is also supplied by the chorda tympani nerve.

The secretomotor fibres to the parotid gland originate from the inferior salivary nucleus. They travel via the glossopharyngeal nerve to the tympanic plexus and then enter the otic ganglion through the lesser petrosal nerve where they synapse and then exit via the auriculotemporal nerve.

Sympathetic nerve fibres, originating from the superior cervical ganglion, pass through the otic ganglion and enter the parotid gland in the auriculotemporal nerve.

In the major salivary glands, parasympathetic nerve stimulation produces a plentiful, fluid saliva, while sympathetic nerve stimulation produces a small quantity of saliva with a high protein content.

The ciliary ganglion

(➲ See Table 12.1)

- Parasympathetic nerve stimulation (causing pupillary constriction) works in opposition to sympathetic nerve stimulation (causing pupillary dilation).
- Parasympathetic nerve fibres from the Edinger–Westphal nucleus pass via the oculomotor nerve to relay in the ciliary ganglion and then innervate the pupil.
- Sympathetic nerves from the superior cervical ganglion pass to the carotid plexus and then travel in the nasociliary nerve to the pupil. An alternative root for the sympathetic nerve supply is for the fibres to pass directly through the ciliary ganglion.

Horner's syndrome

The symptoms arise from damage to the sympathetic nerve supply to the orbit, on the same side as the affected area and include loss of facial sweating, unilateral pupillary constriction, ptosis, and enopthalmos. Ptosis is a drooping of the upper eyelid and enopthalmos is a posterior displacement of the eye.

Acquired ptosis can be an important warning sign of underlying disease affecting the eye, nerves, or muscles and should be investigated. Acquired Horner's syndrome can be caused by trauma, tumours, or vascular disease damaging the sympathetic nerve supply. Given the long sympathetic nerve supply, bronchial carcinoma should be considered in the differential diagnosis. Preganglionic sympathetic fibres reach the superior cervical ganglion from the thoracic spinal cord, synapse and then travel on to the head and neck region.

Argyll–Robertson pupils

In this condition the small pupils do not constrict when light is shone into the eye, but they constrict when viewing near objects (also called a light-near dissociation). It is most likely caused by damage to the midbrain, as midbrain tumours can produce a similar pupillary reaction to that seen with the Argyll–Robertson pupils. The condition is seen in syphilis and diabetes mellitus.

Peripheral autonomic neuropathy

Diabetes

Autonomic neuropathy is caused by damage to the autonomic nerves. It results in:

- Tachycardia (due to vagal damage)
- Nausea and incomplete stomach emptying (gastroparesis)
- Incomplete emptying of the bladder
- Impotence.

Guillain–Barré syndrome

Following an infection, the Guillain–Barré syndrome may result from the immune system attacking the peripheral nervous system. Tachycardia and electrocardiogram (ECG) abnormalities are the most common autonomic abnormalities.

Central autonomic nervous system disorders

Multiple system atrophy (MSA)

This is a neurodegenerative disease affecting the autonomic nervous system. It is associated with either or both degeneration of the striatonigral system (giving atypical parkinsonism) or the olivopontocerebellar system (giving cerebellar ataxia). Affected patients may also present with urinary incontinence and orthostatic hypotension.

Parkinson's disease

Parkinson's disease is associated with mild autonomic dysfunction in the later stages of the disease. One of the main symptoms of this is postural hypotension. There is little evidence that the drooling of saliva is due to excessive production of saliva, rather the opposite is true. A more likely explanation instead is the impaired salivary clearance caused by poor swallowing function.

Vertebrobasilar ischaemia

• May result in paroxysmal hypertension.

Taste sensation

The facial (VII), glossopharyngeal (IX), and vagus nerves (X) supply taste sensation (Table 12.4). The central processes of all three nerves terminate in the nucleus tractus solitarius.

• Palatal taste sensation travels in the greater petrosal nerve, which becomes the nerve of the pterygoid canal. The cell bodies are in the genicular ganglion and central cell processes pass into the sensory root (nervus intermedius). The fibres enter the pons.
• Taste sensation from the anterior tongue is provided by the lingual nerve. Afferent fibres travel in the chorda tympani, and then pass through the sensory root of the facial nerve to the pons.
• The vagus supplies taste sensation to the pharynx.

Table 12.4. Nerves providing taste sensation

Cranial nerve	Nerve branch	Function
Facial nerve	Chorda tympani nerve Greater petrosal nerve	Taste sensation to the anterior two-thirds of the tongue Palatal taste sensation
Glossopharyngeal nerve	Lingual nerve	Taste sensation to the posterior third of the tongue
Vagus nerve	Superior laryngeal nerve	Taste sensation to the epiglottis and pharynx

Trauma to the chorda tympani

The effect of surgical trauma to the chorda tympani is to cause a reduced taste sensation from the anterior two-thirds of the tongue and less salivary flow. If the lingual nerve is also damaged there is a unilateral loss of sensation to the anterior region of the tongue.

Crocodile tears (Bogorad's syndrome)

Tears form during mastication. This occurs as a result of trauma to the facial nerve causing facial paralysis; the regenerating parasympathetic fibres in the facial nerve fibres innervate the tear gland.

Gustatory sweating (Frey's syndrome)

The symptoms of this condition are redness and sweating visible on the cheek near the parotid gland. The syndrome occurs as a result of damage of the auriculotemporal nerve following parotid gland surgery. The sympathetic and parasympathetic nerves that previously innervated the parotid gland now regenerate and innervate the blood vessels and sweat glands of the facial skin.

Modifying patient behaviour

Where the dentist has a good rapport with the patient, then this can have a profound placebo effect on any perception of pain by the patient.

Two techniques can be especially helpful in assisting the patient to cope with the stress of visiting the dentist.

Systematic desensitization

This is the use of counter conditioning which aims to introduce relaxation techniques during exposure to mildly fearful situations. When they have accommodated to the stimulus, the intensity of the stimulus is increased gradually until the most anxiety-provoking stage is reached. During this escalation process, the patient uses relaxation to overcome their anxiety. The technique is successful in treating mild phobias, but not mental disorders.

Modelling

Involves learning by imitation of a positive behaviour. However, the technique has only short-term benefit unless it is reinforced by reward. Therefore, a dentist might suggest a patient watch a simple procedure being performed on an older sibling, to whom the younger child can relate. If the older child is rewarded by encouragement and praise, this provides powerful encouragement for the younger child. If the older child now describes their experience, it can assist the younger child to understand their feelings.

Feedback

Feedback, involving praise, reassurance, and encouragement, is a powerful motivator to encourage positive behavioural change.

The theory of planned behaviour

This theory states that behaviour is determined by external influences and societal norms, but also by an individual's attitude and ability to perform the task.

For example, encouraging a positive attitude in patients towards good oral hygiene would be an important motivator. Demonstrating that they are able to perform effective oral hygiene is also essential.

Transtheoretical model of behavioural change

According to this theory, changing health behaviour involves evolution through several stages of change[1]:

- 'Precontemplation (they do not intend to carry out the change)
- Contemplation (they intend to change)
- Preparation (they have prepared an action plan)
- Action (the change is made)
- Maintenance (to prevent reversion to the old behaviour)
- And termination (the new behaviour is firmly established).

This approach can involve challenging patients to say where they are on the continuum and where they would like to be. The theory allows the clinician to match the intervention to the patient's progress so that it is optimally effective.

The A-B-C model
This describes the following factors as being important in behavioural change (e.g. the features that may be important in improving a patient's oral hygiene):

A Affect
B Behaviour
C Cognition (beliefs)

- A: Affective factors include motivation to change, which are affected by principles and general outlook
- B: Behavioural factors include manual dexterity
- C: Cognition includes the knowledge and attitudes held by the patient.

Self-efficacy
'Self-efficacy' is a term used to describe how confident an individual is at performing a specific task. Those with low self-efficacy are believed not to attempt or persist with tasks where they feel they will fail. In a task designed to improve oral hygiene, self-efficacy in performing the oral hygiene tasks is one of the best predictors of behavioural change. The success of various techniques to motivate change can be assessed by measuring self-efficacy of patients before and after the intervention. However, the patients' self-reported answers will be inaccurate if their replies are designed to be socially acceptable.

Reference
1 Prochaska JO, Velicer WF. (1997) The transtheoretical model of health behavior change. *Amer J Health Promotion* 12:38–48.

Local anaesthesia

How do local anaesthetics work?

Local anaesthetics block the action potential in nerves by preventing sodium ions from entering the cell. They bind to the protein unit of the voltage-gated sodium channels. The local anaesthetic is a weak base, but when injected into the vicinity of the nerve it dissociates into a lipid soluble base which diffuses into the nerve. Inside the nerve, it is the contact of the local anaesthetic with the membrane proteins of the sodium channel that prevents nerve conduction.

The acidic environment surrounding infected tissues may prevent formation of the lipid soluble base and inhibit the nerve block. Most of the commonly used local anaesthetics have amide links between the aromatic ring at one end of the molecule and the amine group at the other, e.g. lidocaine, prilocaine, and articaine. Amides are metabolized by the liver, except articaine where 90–95 % is metabolized in the blood and the remainder by the liver. This is because articaine is classified as an amide due to the amide link, but contains an ester group in the aromatic ring which when it is hydrolysed inactivates the molecule.

Clinical relevance

With local anaesthetics, pain sensation is usually lost before the sense of touch or pressure. Patients may be alarmed that they can still feel the touch and pressure applied by the dentist to a tooth during an extraction. A tooth with acute pulpitis can be difficult to anesthetize. Provided the safe dose is not exceeded, the dentist can overcome this problem by injecting more anaesthetic or combining block anaesthesia and local infiltration techniques.

The duration of anaesthesia is prolonged by incorporating vasopressor agents into many local anaesthetics. Plain lidocaine is a vasodilator and is only suitable for brief dental procedures.

Articaine is metabolized more rapidly than lidocaine, therefore is less toxic. Local buccal infiltration using articaine has been found to have the same efficacy as an inferior alveolar nerve block with lidocaine. This can avoid the discomfort and trismus that can accompany block anaesthesia.

Side-effects of local anaesthetic agents

Overdose

The effect of an overdose of local anaesthetic is to cause convulsive seizures, coma, and respiratory arrest due to the suppression of inhibitory neurones in the CNS.

Side effects can be minimized by:
- Injecting the local anaesthetic slowly
- Avoiding intravascular injection by using an aspiration technique.

Properties of local anaesthetics: maxillary infiltration

The speed of onset and duration of the anaesthesia are partly related to the lipid solubility of the local anaesthetic molecule. (⟳ See Table 12.5) Thus lidocaine and prilocaine with similar lipid solubility have a similar speed of onset of analgesia. Articaine has a slightly lower dissociation constant than

Table 12.5. Local anaesthetics

Local anaesthetic	Onset of anaesthesia	Duration of anaesthesia
2% Lidocaine with 1: 100,000 adrenaline	Rapid onset	~170 minutes
Mepivacaine 3% plain	Rapid onset	~90 minutes
Bupivaciane 0.5% with 1:200,000 adrenaline	Slow onset	Prolonged duration ~ 340 minutes
Prilocaine (4% plain)	Rapid onset	~105 minutes
Articaine(4% with 1:100,000 adrenaline)	Rapid onset	~ 135 minutes*

lidocaine, therefore a greater proportion of the uncharged lipid-soluble molecule will be available in the tissues. Onset of anaesthesia is therefore slightly faster with articaine than lidocaine

Comparison of local anaesthetics

- Differences in the pH of local anaesthetics may be responsible for the finding that buccal infiltrations of bupivacaine cause more pain than prilocaine injections.
- Bupivocaine binds to the protein of the sodium channels with great efficacy, which accounts for the prolonged duration of action.
- Vasopressor agents are used with some local anaesthetics to prolong the duration of contact of the anaesthetic with the nerve and therefore prolong the duration of anaesthesia. Lidocaine, when used by itself, is a vasodilator.[2]

Reference

2 Cowan A. (1977) Clinical assessment of a new local anaesthetic agent: articaine. *Oral Surg Oral Med Oral Pathol* **43**:174–180.

Providing dental local anaesthesia

Procedure for an inferior alveolar nerve block

This is one of the commonest procedures in dentistry. The inferior alveolar nerve is a branch of the posterior branch of the mandibular nerve. It provides a sensory function to the lips, buccal gingivae, and teeth on that side.

The needle enters the mucosa from the premolar region of the opposite side. The syringe is held parallel to the occlusal plane. The injection site is 1 cm above the occlusal plane, between the coronoid process and the pterygomandibular raphe. The needle is advanced about 2–3 cm until resistance is felt as the needle contacts the ramus. The needle is retracted a couple of millimetres. Following aspiration, about 1.5 ml of the local anaesthetic solution is injected slowly. During retraction of the needle the lingual nerve is anaesthetized by depositing 0.5 ml of solution 0.5 cm from the lingula.

When a successful inferior alveolar nerve block has been given, the patient will describe a change in sensation of the lips. The lingual nerve supplies sensory sensation to the anterior two-thirds of the tongue and the lingual gingivae. When the lingual nerve has been anaesthetized the patient will notice a change in sensation of the tongue.

Procedure for a superior alveolar nerve block

A regional block technique should be avoided. Damage to the pterygoid venous plexus is more likely than with the alternative technique where local anaesthetic is infiltrated into the buccal sulcus in the region of the second and third molar teeth.

Infiltration of local anaesthetic in the buccal sulcus of the maxillary third molars requires the patient to half open their mouth so that the cheeks and lips are loose and not tensed. In this position the coronoid process does not obscure the injection site.

The posterior superior alveolar nerve supplies the sensory sensation to the maxillary molar teeth and the mucous membrane of the maxillary sinus. It contributes to a plexus formed by the anterior superior alveolar and the middle superior alveolar nerves

Local complications from an inferior alveolar nerve block

Trismus

- Trismus can arise from needle trauma to the medial pterygoid muscle during the inferior alveolar nerve block. The symptoms usually diminish within a few days.
- Infection can also occur, but is rare.

Facial nerve palsy

This occurs when the local anaesthetic solution is deposited near the posterior ramus of the mandible. The patient is unable to frown.

Damage to the inferior alveolar nerve

Avoid injecting the solution directly into the mental foramen under pressure, otherwise damage to the nerves can result.

Pain
The periosteum of the mandibular ramus should only be lightly touched with the needle during the injection procedure.

Local complications arising from a superior alveolar nerve block

Diplopia
- Arises from a posterior superior alveolar nerve block when the anaesthetic solution is injected too quickly
- The anaesthetic enters the inferior orbital fissure.

Haematoma in the pterygoid venous plexus
This occurs when the needle is advanced too far and damages the pterygoid venous plexus. When the local anaesthetic solution is aspirated, the presence of blood appearing in the cartridge will indicate the leakage of blood into the tissues. The tissues will appear swollen.

Sedation, general anaesthesia, and analgesia

➔ See also Chapter 8

Drugs used in conscious sedation

Some patients request sedation when undergoing a dental procedure. Drugs such as midazolam are anxiolytics used in intravenous sedation. Midazolam is a short-acting benzodiazepine drug. Benzodiazepine agonists potentiate the effect of the inhibitory neurotransmitter GABA. They do this by enhancing the depolarizing effect of GABA by binding to the GABA receptors of the CNS to open chloride ion-selective pores. This increases the neuronal intracellular chloride ion concentration. Benzodiazepines do not activate the GABA receptor directly.

The structure of the various benzodiazepine molecules governs the affinity with which they bind to the GABA receptor and their potency. Lorazepam is a more potent agonist than midazolam, and diazepam is the least potent of the three.

The action of midazolam is reversed by flumazenil which is a benzodiazepine receptor antagonist. Flumazenil is a short-acting drug that is given intravenously.

Clinical relevance

Risks with midazolam sedation are increased in those elderly patients with chronic obstructive pulmonary disease (COPD). The risk is reduced by using a titration regime for people aged 65+ years, which reduces the risk. The half-life of midazolam may be prolonged in those with hepatic or renal dysfunction due to the accumulation of the active metabolite alpha-hydroxy-midazolam. Patients undergoing conscious sedation should be monitored continuously with a pulse oximeter and cardiac monitor to detect early respiratory depression.

General anaesthetics

How do general anaesthetics work?

General anaesthetic agents have a great variety of molecular shape and chemical structure, indicating that they are unlikely to require target receptors with a specific chemical composition. Various hypotheses have been presented to explain the action of general anaesthetics. General anaesthetics bind to ion channels and inhibit their function or they dissolve in the lipid layer of the nerve membrane and exert lateral pressure on the receptor, resulting in ion channel closure.

Propofol (2,6 diisopropylphenol) is used as an intravenous agent to induce general anaesthesia. It is highly lipid soluble with a rapid onset and a brief effect lasting about 15 minutes. It has no analgesic properties and is often combined with the opioid fentanyl. Propofol acts by prolonging the action of the inhibitory neurotransmitter, GABA, at its receptor and increasing the hyperpolarization of the nerve.

General anaesthesia is maintained by oxygen, nitrous oxide, and an inhalation agent such as isoflurane or sevoflurane. The mechanism of action of isoflurane is similar to that of propofol in that there is an enhanced inhibition of neurones; but a different non-receptor mechanism may be responsible. Isoflurane may produce a hyperpolarization in the thalamocortical neurones, mediated by an increased leakage of potassium ions.

Clinical relevance

Sensation, consciousness, and cognitive function depend on the interplay of inhibitory and excitatory neurones. Positron emission tomography scans of volunteers undergoing general anaesthesia have shown that agents such as isoflurane and halothane reduce the metabolic activity of the whole brain, whereas propofol reduces cortical metabolism in a more targeted manner.

The risks assessment of health for those undergoing a general anaesthetic (such as degree of COPD, renal, liver, or other significant co-morbidity) would include use of the ASA (American Society of Anaesthesiologists) score.

Analgesia

It is important to obtain a careful pain history to inform the disease diagnosis. Important factors to consider are:

- To identify the site of the pain
- Its intensity
- Duration
- Quality (sharp, burning, dull ache, etc).

Special care is needed to identify pain in those with dementia as this can be easily missed. Physical signs may include facial grimacing or fist clenching accompanied by hyperventilation and abnormal vocalization (such as groaning and shouting).

The mainstay of pain control in clinical practice is the appropriate use of paracetamol, NSAIDs, and opioids. NSAIDs have an analgesic action due to their inhibition of cyclo-oxygenase enzyme-2 (COX-2) which is induced by inflammation. Note that paracetamol is NOT a NSAID and that codeine is a weak opioid. Fentanyl is an example of a strong opioid. Ibuprofen is a NSAID.

Side-effects of NSAIDs

- Oedema caused by renal impairment
- Prolonged clotting time
- Stomach ulcers
- Can precipitate bronchospasm in those patients with asthma.

Opioid overdose

- Pin-point pupils
- Increased sedation
- Respiratory rate is depressed.

Drug problems in dental practice

Heroin and cocaine use

Amongst those who inject class A drugs, the UK has a high drug-related death rate and high rates of hepatitis C infection. Amongst injecting drug users, the incidence of HIV is low but increasing. There are other associated problems such as shoplifting to fund the drug habit and violence and intimidation underlying the illicit nature of the drug trade. Heroin and crack cocaine use can cause an overdose and both are highly addictive.

Methylenedioxymethamphetamine (MDMA) 'Ecstasy'

MDMA is a sympathomimetic stimulant. Oral symptoms include:
- Dry mouth and if carbonated drinks are used this can produce tooth erosion; sugary drinks increase the risk of caries
- Bruxism and jaw clenching
- Dental attrition, due to clenching, vomiting, and the absence of buffering saliva
- Lip paraesthesia, especially with high doses.

Systemic side-effects include liver damage, psychiatric disorder, tachycardia, raised body temperature, and pupillary dilation. In users of MDMA, there may be damage to brain serotonin (5-HT) neurons which may explain the reported loss of short-term memory. Tiredness is often reported a day or two after taking the drug.

MDMA stimulates the secretion of antidiuretic hormone which prevents the excretion of the fluid consumed as a result of the xerostomia. This may be potentially life-threatening, resulting in hyponatraemia, cerebral oedema, and unconsciousness.

Alcohol

See also ➲ Alcohol and the dental patient in Chapter 5.

The UK Chief Medical Officers' guideline for men and women is that they drink regularly no more than 14 units a week (which is equivalent to about 6 pints of 4% beer or 6 glasses of 13% wine). The risk of mouth cancer increases with increasing alcohol consumption on a regular basis.

Excessive alcohol consumption can cause general complications such as:
- Liver cirrhosis
- Chronic pancreatitis
- Intracerebral haemorrhage
- Foetal alcohol spectrum disorder.

Oral complications include:
- Oral cancer
- Dry mouth
- Sialosis (enlargement of the major salivary glands).

Alcoholics may also have an increased risk of caries, and periodontal disease as a result of self-neglect. Dental erosion may result from regular vomiting.

Tobacco smoking

Smoking causes oral squamous cell carcinoma and has a multiplicative effect if combined with large quantities of alcoholic spirits. Chewing smokeless tobacco (e.g. combined with areca nut in a betel quid) is also a risk factor for oral cancer.

Smoking tobacco also increases the risk of periodontal bone loss but there is usually less gingival bleeding observed. Treatment of periodontal disease, whether surgical or non-surgical, is also less effective. There is overwhelming evidence for a benefit to healthcare professionals advising patients to stop smoking.

Prescribing drugs for children

Prescribing drugs for children has some important considerations:
• Tetracycline can cause staining of developing teeth
• Avoid aspirin and other non-steroidal anti-inflammatory drugs because of the possibility of causing Reye's syndrome (manifested as liver and brain damage).

Common drug interactions

• Adrenaline-containing local anaesthetic may interact with beta-adrenoreceptor blocking drugs to increase the patient's hypertension. This is due to adrenaline causing peripheral vasoconstriction and a tachycardia. It is advised to use a limited amount of adrenaline-containing local anaesthetic (3 cartridges) or use an adrenaline-free local anesthetic.
• Warfarin can interact with miconazole, metronidazole, and erythromycin to cause excessive bleeding.

Side-effects of drugs used in sedation

Nitrous oxide
Used in inhalation sedation.
• Inactivates vitamin B_{12} by causing irreversible oxidation of the cobalt ion. Methylation of myelin phospholipids is prevented which inhibits myelin formation. Myeloneuropathy and subacute combined degeneration of the spinal cord results from long-term abuse of nitrous oxide.
• Increased risk of congenital abnormalities with prolonged exposure.

Benzodiazepines
They facilitate the binding of GABA to the receptor site, which mediates inhibitory impulses in the CNS.
Side-effects include:
• Respiratory depression with rapid intra-venous injection
• Impairment of memory storage and anterograde amnesia
• Physical dependence with long-term use.

Dementia

This is a major disease entity and its rising incidence follows the increasing life expectancy of the population.
    Forms of dementia include:
- Lewy body disease
- Vascular dementia
- Hippocampal sclerosis
- Fronto-temporal lobe degeneration and dementia
- Alzheimer's disease.

Alzheimer's disease

The symptoms increase gradually in severity as the disease is insidious in onset. Those mildly affected complain of memory loss, but the symptoms increase in severity resulting in confusion and delusions, and the later stages involve speech loss, urinary incontinence, and difficulty in eating.
    The symptoms result from the death of neurons in the CNS caused by the accumulation of amyloid beta to form amyloid plaques.
    Alzheimer's disease has two variations: a genetically inherited and a sporadic form. (➲ See Table 12.6)

Dyskinesia

Some neuroleptic drugs induce involuntary tongue and jaw movements which can make denture wearing extremely difficult. This movement disorder is called tardive dyskinesia and is due to the blockage of dopamine receptors in the CNS by dopamine antagonists. Dyskinesia is a disorder where the patient suffers involuntary muscle movements. Different types are known:

Dystonia

This is a continuous muscle spasm due to disease of the basal ganglia or antipsychotic drugs.

Table 12.6. Classification of Alzheimer's disease

	Familial Alzheimer's disease	Sporadic form of Alzheimer's disease
Onset	About 40 years	Over 60 years
Cause	Genetic	Genetic and environmental causes
Prevalence	Uncommon form	More common form

Tardive dyskinesia
Typically results from long-term use of antipsychotic drugs.

Levodopa-induced dyskinesia
This condition may be observed in patients with Parkinson's disease who have been receiving levodopa (L-DOPA) for long periods.

Clinical relevance

Dental care for those with dementia
Patients with dementia may be receiving antidepressant drugs which reduce salivation and increase the risk of caries and periodontal disease. By applying fluoride varnishes to the teeth and prescribing high concentration fluoride toothpaste, the dentist can help to prevent caries. The dentist or hygienist should instruct the patient and carer in oral hygiene methods and encourage twice daily brushing, in the morning and in the evening. An electric toothbrush can be very helpful in maintaining an adequate oral hygiene.

Denture wearing
The lack of salivary lubrication can reduce a patient's ability to wear dentures. Denture adhesives, applied to the fitting surface of the denture, can assist in denture retention. In a nursing home environment, dentures can be lost and the patient's memory loss can increase the likelihood of this happening. The dentist can mark the dentures with the patient's initials so that if they should be mislaid they can be quickly returned to the patient.

Complete denture wearing in patients with dementia or tardive dyskinesia can be difficult. When a new denture is needed, it may be possible to copy many of the features of the patient's existing dentures but improve the retention and occlusion. By preserving some aspects of the denture shape, the patient may be able to adapt to the denture much more easily.

Chapter 13

Endocrine system

Reproductive hormones and their function 288
Gastrointestinal hormones and their function 292
Skeletal hormones 294
The adrenal gland 296
The thyroid gland 298
Growth hormones 302

Reproductive hormones and their function

Female reproductive hormones

The hypothalamus secretes gonadotropin-releasing hormone which stimulates the anterior pituitary to release luteinizing hormone (LH) and follicle stimulating hormone (FSH). Oestrogen is released by the ovary and its regulation is governed by FSH.

The menstrual cycle

The menstrual cycle can be divided into two phases; the follicular phase (0–14 days of the cycle) and the luteal phase (14–28 days). About 2 days before the onset of menstruation, there is a rise in FSH release which stimulates growth of about 6–10 follicles in the ovary. The follicles produce oestrogen which has a negative feedback effect on the pituitary causing a decrease in FSH secretion. However, increasing LH levels are seen throughout the follicular phase. The declining levels of FSH cause follicular atresia, with the continued survival of only one dominant follicle. This follicle continues to produce oestrogen until a trigger point is reached, with positive feedback causing a mid-cycle LH surge (dotted line in Fig. 13.1).

In the ovary, the LH surge causes ovulation and the ruptured follicle develops to form the corpus luteum. Progesterone and oestrogen are produced by the corpus luteum and this phase after ovulation is called the luteal phase. Progesterone prepares the endometrium for implantation of the blastocyst.

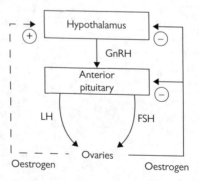

GnRH = Gonadotropin releasing homone

FSH = Follicle-stimulating hormone

LH = Luteinizing hormone

Fig. 13.1 Interaction between the ovaries, pituitary and hypothalamus produces the menstrual cycle.

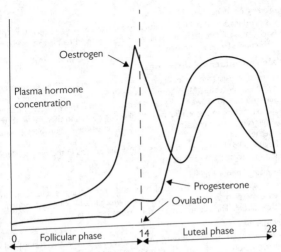

Fig. 13.2 Changes in the concentration of plasma oestrogen and progesterone during the menstrual cycle.

If implantation does not occur, declining levels of oestrogen, inhibin A, and progesterone cause FSH levels to rise and menstruation begins a few days later. (➲ See Fig. 13.2)

Oestrogen
Oestrogen is the family name for a group of hormones involved in female sexual development and in the menstrual cycle. Oestrogen is given as a component of some oral contraceptive therapies and in oestrogen replacement therapy for peri-menopausal and postmenopausal women.

Follicle stimulating hormone (FSH)
FSH and LH act synergistically in women. FSH stimulates the development of the ovarian follicles (follicular phase) and the cells start to produce increasing amounts of oestradiol and inhibin. Inhibin prevents FSH synthesis and secretion.

Inhibin
Inhibin A and B are produced by the ovary. Inhibin B inhibits the secretion of FSH during the follicular phase. Inhibin A may reduce secretion of FSH in the luteal phase.

Progesterone
In the follicular phase, serum progesterone levels remain low up until the LH-surge. The increasing serum concentration of progesterone terminates the LH-surge. The corpus luteum produces progesterone.

Luteinizing hormone (LH)

LH is produced by the anterior pituitary cells and a surge in secretion triggers ovulation. Detection of urinary LH can be used to predict ovulation and the period when a woman can become pregnant.

Male reproductive hormones

Spermatogenesis (the production of sperm) occurs in the seminiferous tubules of the testes. Male germ cells are present on the outside of the tubule and develop towards the centre, maturing into spermatids. The spermatozoa mature in the epididymis, a collecting duct, and then move to the vas deferens. The prostate gland and seminal vesicles contribute fluid to the semen.

Leydig cells lie adjacent to the seminiferous tubules in the testicle. Their function is to secrete testosterone.

Luteinizing hormone (LH)

LH is produced in the hypothalamus and stimulates the secretion and release of testosterone from Leydig cells which in turn inhibits the further release of LH. This is an example of negative feedback.

Testosterone

Testosterone is mainly produced by the Leydig cells in the testis (and a minor fraction by the adrenal cortex). Testosterone has a local regulatory effect on the Sertoli cells which nourish the spermatozoa. With age there is a gradual decrease in testosterone secretion by the testis which may contribute to a decreased muscle volume and bone density.

Gonadotrophin-releasing hormone (GnRH)

GnRH is a hypothalamic factor that controls the release of LH and FSH from the anterior pituitary. GnRH is released in a pulsatile manner when testosterone levels are low, thereby stimulating the pituitary to release LH. This stimulates the Leydig cells in the testicles to secrete testosterone which has a negative effect on the further release of GnRH.

Follicle stimulating hormone (FSH)

FSH stimulates spermatogenesis. FSH controls the function of Sertoli cells which are in close contact with the spermatids as they develop.

Inhibin

Inhibin has a negative feedback effect on the secretion of FSH.

Gastrointestinal hormones and their function

See also ➲ Digestive tract in Chapter 1.

Gastrin

Gastrin is synthesized in the G-cells, present in the distal part of the stomach and the initial part of the duodenum. Its function is to stimulate gastric acid secretion and gastric and small intestinal motility.

Cholecystokinin

Cholecystokinin is produced by the I cells in the mucosa of the duodenum. Cholecystokinin stimulates gall bladder contraction, and enzyme, insulin, and glucagon secretion in the pancreas. When given exogenously, it inhibits gastric emptying by causing the pyloric sphincter to contract.

Secretin

Secretin is produced by the S-cells of the duodenum and jejunum and stimulates the production of an alkaline pancreatic fluid when the pH of the duodenum becomes less than 4.5. There are several other members of the secretin family (e.g. glucose-dependent insulinotropic peptide, glucagon, and vasoactive intestinal peptide).

Ghrelin

This hormone stimulates increased food intake and the deposition of adipose tissue. It is produced by the stomach. The fasting serum level of ghrelin is inversely related to BMI with raised levels in those with anorexia nervosa.

Peptide tyrosine tyrosine (PYY)

This peptide is released from the intestine following a meal and slows the intestinal transit of food through the intestine. In obese patients, PYY reduces body weight by inducing satiety.

Neuropeptide Y

Neuropeptide Y is a neurotransmitter located mainly in the upper intestine and distal colon. It causes vasoconstriction and reduced intestinal secretion.

Somatostatin

Somatostatin is secreted by D cells in the gut mucosa. Its release is stimulated by fatty and proteinaceous food. It inhibits a wide spectrum of GI functions: secretion of several gut hormones, gastric acid, and pancreatic enzymes; gastric emptying; and absorption of some nutrients, such as amino acids and fat in the small intestine.

Vasoactive intestinal peptide (VIP)

VIP is a neurotransmitter that reduces gastric secretion.

Obesity

The action of the GI hormones on the hypothalamus and brain stem is important in determining food intake. (➲ See Table 13.1)

Table 13.1 GI hormones

Hormones stimulating appetite	Hormones stimulating satiety
Ghrelin	PYY
	Cholecystokinin
	GLP
	Pancreatic polypeptide
	Oxyntomodulin

Ghrelin is the only known hormone to stimulate appetite. In obese individuals there is lack of suppression of ghrelin levels following a meal. Dieting alone can be unsuccessful in a weight loss programme because it causes an increase in ghrelin secretion which stimulates a desire for food.

Glucagon-like peptide-1 (GLP-1) and glucose-dependent insulinotropic polypeptide (GIP) are incretin peptides that stimulate insulin secretion from the pancreas following a meal. GLP-1inhibits gastric emptying. Oxyntomodulin is synthesized by cells in the intestine and colon, and together with the incretin peptides and PYY, causes satiety by delaying gastric emptying. Pancreatic polypeptide is secreted by the islets of Langerhans according to the calorific value of the food intake and functions to reduce further food ingestion.

The effect of bariatric surgery on GI hormones

Bariatric surgery is an effective method of inducing significant weight loss. Gastric bypass procedures cause increased plasma PYY and GLP-1 following a meal, which induce a reduced food intake and satiety[1].

Do GI hormones play a role in obesity?

Obesity may result from an exaggerated brain response to the anticipation of food and a decreased response when the food is consumed. Obese patients may consume more food in an attempt to compensate for the reduced reward. GLP-1 may be an important gastro-endocrine hormone regulating the reward experienced by the anticipation and consumption of food has the effect of inducing satiety. When GLP-1 receptor agonists, e.g. exenatide are given, then there is an increased brain response to the consumption of food which leads to a reduced food consumption[2].

References

1. le Roux CW, Aylwin SJ, Batterham RL, Borg CM, Coyle F, Prasad V, Shurey S, Ghatei MA, Patel AG, Bloom SR. (2006) Gut hormone profiles following bariatric surgery favor an anorectic state, facilitate weight loss, and improve metabolic parameters. *Ann Surg* 243:108–14.
2. van Bloemendaal L, Veltman DJ, Ten Kulve JS, Groot PF, Ruhé HG, Barkhof F, Sloan JH, Diamant M, IJzerman RG. (2015) Brain reward-system activation in response to anticipation and consumption of palatable food is altered by GLP-1 receptor activation in humans. *Diabetes Obes Metab* 17: 878–86.

Skeletal hormones

See also $\bigcirc$ Bone in Chapter 4.

Parathyroid hormone

Extracellular calcium ion concentration is sensed by a membrane protein on the surface of the parathyroid cells which controls the synthesis and secretion of parathyroid hormone. This hormone increases renal calcium reabsorption and phosphate excretion.

1,25 hydroxyvitamin D_3

The main hormones acting on bone are parathyroid hormone and 1,25 hydroxyvitamin D_3. Parathyroid hormone increases the conversion of 25-hydroxyvitamin D to the active metabolite 1,25 hydroxyvitamin D_3 in the kidney and also increases bone resorption. 1,25 hydroxyvitamin D_3 increases the absorption of calcium from the gut.

Control of bone resorption

Bone resorption is initiated by the fusion of osteoclast precursor cells to form osteoclasts. Osteoclasts resorb bone. Cells of the osteoblast lineage express RANK ligand (RANKL) which is necessary for osteoclast differentiation. RANKL binds to its receptor RANK on the surface of the osteoclast precursor and initiates osteoclast differentiation. Osteoprotogerin opposes this effect on osteoclast differentiation. It is the ratio between osteoprotogerin and RANKL in the bone marrow environment which determines whether osteoclast differentiation takes place.

In periodontal disease, RANKL is expressed by activated lymphocytes as well as stromal cells. Cells expressing cytokines can influence bone resorption by stimulating the differentiation of osteoclasts.

Mechanism of bone resorption

Osteoclasts form resorption lacunae (called Howship's lacunae) on the bone surface. They arise from haematopoietic progenitor cells whereas osteoblasts differentiate from mesenchymal stem cells. Osteoblasts, which are involved in bone formation, also control osteoclast differentiation. The balance in bone formation and resorption is controlled by a range of hormones and growth factors acting on the stromal cells.

The process of bone resorption has the following steps:
* The osteoblast removes surface osteoid.
* The osteoclast attaches to the bone surface and forms an extracellular demineralizing zone enclosed by the ruffled border. The osteoclast removes organic matrix by releasing cathepsins.
* The activity of the osteoclast ceases and is followed by deposition of bone by the osteoblast.

Mechanism of bone formation

Bone formation occurs by the maturation of osteoprogenitor cells to pre-osteoblasts and osteoblasts. These cells express a variety of bone matrix proteins as they mature. Some of the osteoblasts become trapped in the secreted osteoid and form osteocytes. The osteocytes are in direct contact with the surface cell layer despite being entombed in the calcified matrix.

Orthodontic tooth movement

Orthodontic movement occurs when a continuous light force is applied to one side of a tooth. There is a balance between alveolar bone resorption and deposition. Osteocytes probably provide a mechano-sensing role, by detecting deformation of alveolar bone by the orthodontic force. This results in the differential recruitment of osteoclasts and osteoblasts. Compression of the periodontal ligament causes an avascular necrosis (or focal hyalinization) which up-regulates expression of RANKL. Osteoclasts are recruited to resorb the bone and necrotic periodontal ligament. Until this takes place, no tooth movement can occur.

On the tension side of the tooth, bone deposition occurs through recruitment of osteoblasts. Excessive orthodontic force can cause tooth resorption or ankylosis.

Excessive bone resorption

Menopause

Following the menopause, there is an increased expression of RANKL in bone marrow cells leading to an imbalance in bone turnover and increased bone resorption. Postmenopausal osteoporosis is characterized by an increased risk of fractures of the hip, wrist, and vertebrae.

Primary hyperparathyroidism

Primary hyperparathyroidism is defined by excessive secretion of parathyroid hormone by the parathyroid glands. This stimulates augmented osteoclastic activity with increased serum calcium, but a low or normal serum phosphate level. The patient may develop kidney stones. Bone resorption is observed on radiographs and on skull radiographs it is described as a 'salt and pepper' appearance. This appearance is caused by many small areas of radiolucency following trabecular bone resorption.

Insufficient bone resorption

Osteopetrosis

Osteopetrosis is caused by an inability of the osteoclasts to resorb bone. There is bone fragility despite the increased bone density. In the severest form of the disease with the poorest prognosis, i.e. when diagnosed in infancy, there is usually bone marrow failure and anaemia. This is due to obliteration of the bone marrow cavity. Early haematopoietic stem cell transplantation should be considered in treatment. Even less severely affected individuals may suffer compression of cranial nerves with the optic, trigeminal, and facial nerves affected. Chronic osteomyelitis may result from a tooth extraction as there is reduced bone vascularity.

The adrenal gland

Anatomy

The adrenal glands lie above the kidneys and below the diaphragm. The gland is composed of an outer cortex surrounding an inner medulla. The medulla synthesizes catecholamines and the cortex secretes steroids (glucocorticoids and mineralocorticoids). (➲ See Fig. 13.3)

Corticotrophin-releasing hormone is produced by the hypothalamus in response to stress and stimulates the release of adrenocorticotrophic hormone (ACTH) from the anterior pituitary. ACTH stimulates the release of cortisol from the adrenal gland which has an inhibitory effect on the hypothalamus and pituitary and thereby prevents any further increase in serum cortisol. A deficiency of production of cortisol by the adrenal glands causes Addison's disease whereas an excess production of cortisol from the adrenal gland results in endogenous Cushing's syndrome.

Cushing's syndrome

In endogenous Cushing's syndrome, the excess corticol causes insulin resistance, a reduced secretion of insulin, and hyperglycaemia. Wasting of the proximal muscles occurs through the inhibition of protein muscle synthesis and the activation of muscle proteolysis. Low-dose inhaled corticosteroids are not usually associated with myopathy as a side-effect.

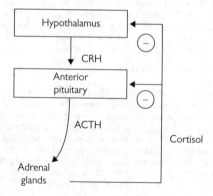

CRH = Corticotrophin releasing hormone
TRH = Adrenocortrophic hormone

Fig. 13.3 Regulation of cortisol concentration in the blood.

Table 13.2 The systemic effects of a deficiency of cortisol production (Addison's disease) compared with an excess production (endogenous Cushing's syndrome)

Addison's disease	Endogenous Cushing's syndrome
Muscle weakness	Muscle weakness
Weight loss	Weight gain
Low blood pressure	Hypertension
Hypoglycaemia	Hyperglycaemia and diabetes

The administration of glucocorticoids can cause exogenous Cushing's syndrome (Table 13.2). The excess corticosteroid will suppress secretion of ACTH, causing adrenal atrophy. If the exogenous corticosteroid medication is stopped, this can precipitate adrenal insufficiency and adrenal crisis if the patient is faced with stress or infection. Patients who are taking or have taken corticosteroids in the previous year should therefore be considered for hydrocortisone supplementation prior to surgery.

The thyroid gland

Anatomy

The thyroid gland lies below and to either side of the larynx with the right and left lobes connected by a narrow isthmus. The parathyroid glands are smaller (about 6 mm in length) and lie on the posterior border of the thyroid gland. The cells of the thyroid gland are filled with thyroglobulin which can be converted to thyroxine and triiodothyronine and released into the circulation. The thyroid gland also contains parafollicular cells which synthesize calcitonin which inhibits osteoclastic resorption of bone.

Decreased serum levels of thyroid hormone stimulates the hypothalamus to release thyrotrophin releasing hormone (TRH) which causes release of thyroid stimulating hormone (TSH) from the anterior pituitary. TSH binds to receptors on the thyroid gland, resulting in release of the thyroid hormones to restore the normal serum concentration. Thyrotoxicosis occurs when there is an excessive circulating level of thyroid hormones. Hypothyroidism is a decreased serum level of thyroid hormones and can result from abnormalities in the pituitary, hypothalamus, or thyroid gland. However, it is most commonly the result of a deficiency of iodine in the diet. Myxoedema occurs in older children and adults. (➲ See Fig. 13.4)

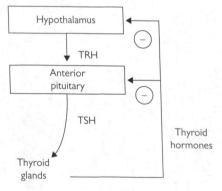

TSH = Thyroid-stimulating hormone

TRH = Thyrotropin-releasing hormone

Fig. 13.4 Regulation of serum thyroid hormone level.

Role of thyroxine

Thyroxine regulates the body's metabolic rate. This explains the lassitude observed in hypothyroidism and the weight loss commonly observed in hyperthyroidism.

Release of T3 and T4

TSH stimulates the release of T3 and T4 from thyroglobulin.

Transport of thyroxine

Following release from the thyroid glands, thyroxine (T4) and 3-5,3'-triiodothyronine (T3) are transported to the target cells by carrier proteins, mainly thyroxine-binding globulin (TBG).

Thyroxine (T4) and 3-5,3'-triiodothyronine (T3) activity

T4 is a prohormone with minimal effect as it is converted to T3 (the active hormone) as required in the tissues. This conversion is catalysed by iodo-thyronine deiodinase and the rate is determined by the uptake of T3 and T4 into the cells.

Triiodothyronine acts on nuclear thyroid hormone receptors in the cell. In turn, these receptors interact with genes responsive to that hormone. The resulting effect of the interaction between the T3 binding to the receptor and the gene is changes in the cell mRNA levels and increased or decreased concentrations of proteins. T3 has a variety of different tissue-specific effects. (➲ See Fig. 13.5)

Both hyperthyroidism and hypothyroidism may be associated with goitre or enlargement of the thyroid gland. (➲ See Table 13.3)

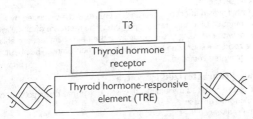

Fig. 13.5 T3 acts on thyroid hormone receptors which regulate gene expression by binding to thyroid hormone response elements (TRE) in DNA. Binding of the T3-thyroid hormone receptor complex to the TRE activates transcription.

Table 13.3 Clinical features comparing hypo- and hyperthyroidism

Hyperthyroidism	Hypothyroidism
Increased metabolic rate	Intolerant of the cold
Increased cardiac output	Reduced cardiac output
Other symptoms	
Ocular changes – appearance of 'bulging' eyes	Tongue enlargement
Muscular atrophy	Coarse skin

Hyperthyroidism

This occurs as a result of too high a circulating level of thyroid hormones. In Graves' disease, hyperthyroidism results from autoantibodies to the TSH receptors which stimulate the unregulated production of thyroid hormone.

Toxic adenoma and multinodular toxic goitre also cause hyperthyroidism and occur more commonly in areas of iodine deficiency. They are slowly growing goitres which function independently of TSH to produce increased levels of thyroid hormones. In hyperthyroidism, the levels of TSH are usually low (<0.1 milli-International Units per ml).

Hypothyroidism

If nonthyroid disease is absent, low thyroxine and increased TSH levels are diagnostic of hypothyroidism. This is a result of the feedback loops previously described where the increased TSH is produced to encourage further thyroxine secretion.

Hypothyroidism affecting children (cretinism) is characterized by a large tongue often causing an anterior open bite. The teeth are often delayed in eruption, with crowding in the small jaws; the pulp chambers are enlarged and the roots are short due to delayed dentine deposition. The physical and mental growth is retarded.

Diseases characterized by goitre

A goitre is an enlarged thyroid gland. Disease that may cause goitre include:
• Hashimoto's disease
• Graves' disease
• Iodine deficiency: not seen in developed countries where salt is iodized.
• Multinodular goitre
• Pregnancy: caused by human chorionic gonadotropin.
• Thyroid cancer.

Hashimoto's Disease

This is an autoimmune disease, i.e. where the body's immune system produces antibodies against the patient's own proteins. In this case, the antibodies are produced against thyroglobulin and thyroid peroxidase. Thyroid peroxidase has the role in the thyroid follicular cell of converting iodide to iodine which is then incorporated into thyroglobulin.

An enlarged thyroid is common in Hashimoto's thyroiditis.

A recent meta-analysis[1] has shown an association between papillary thyroid carcinoma (PTC) and Hashimoto's disease. Therefore, patients with Hashimoto's disease should be assessed regularly for the development of papillary thyroid carcinoma[1].

Multinodular goitre (MNG)

The enlarged thyroid in multinodular goitre has numerous enlarged lumps. The goitre can be either non-toxic MNG (where the circulating thyroid hormone level is normal) or toxic MNG (where the thyroid hormone levels are increased).

Ultrasound is a good technique for assessing the extension of the MNG and the size of the nodules. The cause of MNG is multifactorial. It is prudent to recommend an enlarged thyroid gland be regularly assessed, even where this is symptomless. This would exclude thyroid cancer.

Thyroid cancer

This is a rare form of cancer, accounting for less than 1% of all cancers in the UK.

There are four types of thyroid cancer:
- Papillary carcinoma
- Follicular carcinoma
- Medullary thyroid carcinoma
- Anaplastic thyroid carcinoma.

In general, papillary and follicular cancers have the better prognosis, with 95% survival over 10 years for papillary carcinomas and 90% for follicular carcinomas. In medullary thyroid carcinoma, prognosis is reasonably good (75% survival over 10 years), but those with anaplastic carcinomas have the worst prognosis (15% survival over 10 years).

Reference

[3] Lee JH, Kim Y, Choi JW, Kim YS. (2013) The association between papillary thyroid carcinoma and histologically proven Hashimoto's thyroiditis: a meta-analysis. *Eur J Endocrinol* **168**:343–9.

Growth hormones

Growth hormone is the main hormone that stimulates body growth.

Release of growth hormone from the anterior pituitary is regulated by neurons in the hypothalamus. Growth hormone release is stimulated by growth hormone releasing hormone (GHRH) and inhibited by somatostatin. (➲ See Fig. 13.6)

Insulin-like growth factor is produced in the liver under the influence of growth hormone and is the main intermediary hormone in causing growth. Circulating insulin-like growth factor inhibits growth hormone secretion in a negative feedback fashion.

Somatostatin, produced locally in the tissue, also inhibits the secretion of

- Insulin and glucagon from the pancreas
- Cholecystokinin, vasoactive intestinal polypeptide, gastrin, and secretin in the gastrointestinal tract. The effect is to inhibit various functions of the gastrointestinal tract, e.g. release of stomach acid and digestive enzymes.

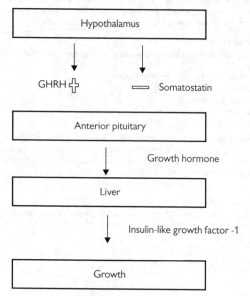

Fig. 13.6 Regulation of growth hormone.

Abnormalities of growth hormone

Excess circulating growth hormone, produced by pituitary adenomas in the adult, causes acromegaly. This condition is characterized by

- Continuous enlargement of the head, hands and feet
- Frontal bossing (forehead prominence) and prominent cheek bones
- Fingers are wider
- Spacing of the teeth
- Maxillary widening and a prognathic mandible
- Skin thickening due to excessive deposition of collagen
- Hypertension
- Insulin resistance, hyperinsulinaemia, and diabetes mellitus

Excess circulating growth hormone in children causes pituitary gigantism. This is characterized by extreme growth of the skeleton, because the long bone epiphyses have not fused, with general enlargement of the organs. It is a rare condition, with excessive secretion of GHRH as an important aetiological factor.

Actions of growth hormone and insulin-like growth factor

At the growth plate

Growth at the epiphyseal plate is controlled closely by the integrated action of paracrine factors and numerous hormones; such as growth hormone, insulin-like growth factor, thyroxine, glucocorticoids, testosterone, and oestrogen. Growth hormone may also act directly on the growth plate chondrocytes and therefore affect growth in a manner independent of insulin-like growth factor.

Action of growth hormone on muscle

Growth hormone is widely abused as a performance-enhancing agent, often in regimes involving combinations of anabolic steroids, insulin-like growth factor, or insulin. Insulin and insulin-like growth factor can both cause severe hypoglycaemia.

Growth hormone has an anabolic effect in muscle by stimulating protein synthesis. It has its anabolic effects by acting directly on muscle as well as stimulating circulating and locally induced insulin-like growth factor.

Index

Note: Tables and figures are indicated by an italic *t* and *f* following the page number.

A

A-B-C model of behavioural change 275
abciximab 224
abdominal aortic aneurysms 203
abducent nerve nerve (cranial nerve VI) 267
abscess formation 244
absorption
  carbohydrates 35
  fat 34
  minerals 35
  protein 34
  vitamins 35
abuse 222–4
acenocoumarol 224
acetaminophen see paracetamol
acetylcholine 62
aciclovir 139
acquired pellicle 23
acromegaly 303
Actinomyces 250
  naelundii 23
  odontolyticus 23
  viscosus 98
action potential 258–9
activated partial thromboplastin time (APTT) 221
  coagulation screen 221
acute phase response 248
Addison's disease 248, 296, 297
adrenal gland 296–7
  anatomy 296
  cortisol regulation 296
adrenaline (epinephrine)
  biotransformation in local anaesthetic 269
  cardiovascular disease 200
  contraindicated in stroke patients 204
  heart failure 198–9
  implanted devices 199
  hypersensitivity 246
adrenergic neurotransmitters 269
adrenocorticotrophic hormone (ACTH) 296
  Cushing's syndrome 297

advanced glycation end products (AGEs) 152
aerosols
  as cause of disease 183
  fate 255
  infection control 255
age factors
  asthma 180
  bone 106
  chronic obstructive pulmonary disease 180
  diabetic retinopathy 160–1
  drug metabolism in the liver 117
  leukaemia 226–7
  myocardial infarction 197
  obstructive sleep apnoea 178–9
  stroke 204–5
  see also children; elderly patients
ageing process
  nerve and muscle function 60–1
  testosterone secretion 290
agglutinogens 228
Aggregatibacter actinomycetemcomitans 203
AIDS see HIV/AIDS
airborne particles, fate of 255
alanine aminotransferase (ALT) 128
albumin 128
alcohol 120–1
  abuse 120–1, 282
  dental care 130
  inhalation of dentures 177
  obstructive sleep apnoea 178–9
  dependence 121
  excess intake, clues to 120–1
  liver disease 122
    complications 122–3
  oral cancer 106–7
  oral mucosa, effect on 71–2
  potential harms 120–1
  recommendations 120, 282
  screening patients 120
aldosterone 135, 137
aldosterone antagonists 199

alkaline phosphatase (ALP) 128
allergies 246
allodynia 262
allografts 96
alteplase 224
alveolar clefts 101
alveolar osteitis ('dry socket') 98–9
  pathogenesis 98
  predisposing conditions 99
  prevention 99
  treatment 99
alveoli 170
  control of respiratory exchange 172–3
  macrophages 235
  physiological dead space 171
  respiratory drive 171
Alzheimer's disease 284
  classification 284
amelo-dentinal junction (ADJ) 14
American Society of Anesthesiologists classifications 184, 281
amino acids 34
amitriptyline 269
amlodipine 200
amoxicillin 139, 168, 224
amphotericin 139
amylase 150
anaemia 216–19
  causes 217
  chronic kidney disease 148
  chronic renal failure 142–3, 146
  clinical relevance 219
  drug causes 219
  gas exchange 170
  haemolytic 247
  oral mucosa, effect on 71–2
  pernicious 248
  types 217
  white blood cells, malignancy of 227
anaesthesia 184–5
  see also general anaesthesia; local anaesthesia
analgesia 281
  impaired liver function, patients with 131

anaphylaxis
drug reactions 246, 247
gas exchange 170
anaplastic thyroid
carcinoma 301
anatomic dead space
(ADS) 175
angina 196–7
clinical relevance 197
referred pain 269
angiotensin-converting
enzyme (ACE)
inhibitors
cardiovascular disease 200
chronic renal
failure 138–9
heart failure 199
renovascular
hypertension 141
angiotensin receptor
blockers (ARB) 199
angular cheilitis 163
anorexia nervosa 36
pancreatic
polypeptide 150–1
anterior (incisal)
guidance 54–5
anterior repositioning
splint 51
anterior superior alveolar
nerve 265
antibiotics
chronic renal failure 139
diabetes 168
hypersensitivity to 246
impaired liver function,
patients with 131
infective endocarditis 202
rheumatic fever 202
and warfarin, interaction
between 200
antibodies 115
actions 237
structure 236
types 236–7
anticholinergic drugs 269
anticoagulants 224
atrial fibrillation 192
infective endocarditis,
patients at risk of 203
stroke patients 204
antidiuretic hormone
(vasopressin) 135, 137
MDMA (ecstasy) 282
antifungals 131
antigen presenting cells
(APCs) 240
antigens 228
destruction 237
immunization 238
antihypertensive drugs 194
antiplatelet medication 224

antiseptic mouth rinses
alveolar osteitis,
prevention of 98, 99
extraction socket 98, 99
apex locators 199
aphasia 82
clinical application 83–4
apixaban 200, 224
aplastic anaemia 219
apneustic centre 173
apoptosis 70
diabetes 160–1
appetite 34–5
Argyll–Robertson pupils 271
arrhythmias 192
cardiovascular implantable
electronic devices 199
arthritis 247
rheumatoid 248
articaine 276–7
articular disc
lateral pterygoid
muscle 45
temporomandibular
joint 48, 50–1
disorders 50, 51
articulation 82–4
articulators 55
ascites 122
aspartate aminotransferase
(AST) 128
aspiration pneumonia 78
stroke patients 204
aspirin
allergy 182
anaemia 219
asthma 182, 183
binding with plasma
proteins 116
blood clotting
impairment 224
contraindicated in
children 283
Reye's syndrome 126, 283
transient ischaemic
attack 205
asthma 181–2
age factors 180
attacks
precipitants 183
recognition 182
FEV1 and FVC 174
atenolol 200
atherosclerosis 196–7
oral bacteria 203
atorvastatin 200
atrial fibrillation 192
atrial natriuretic hormone
(ANP) 137
atrioventricular (AV)
node 191
arrhythmias 192

atrophic candidiasis,
chronic 163
AUDIT (C) 120
auriculotemporal nerve 270
trauma 273
autografts 96
autoimmune
disease 234, 248
Hashimoto's disease 301
autoinducers 250–1
automatic defibrillators 199
autonomic nervous
system 268–73
anatomy in head and neck
region 269, 270
pharmacology 269

B

B lymphocytes 208,
210, 234
cell-mediated
response 240
humoral response 235–6
types 235
bacteraemia 203
infective
endocarditis 202, 203
bacteria, oral 250
bacterial sialadenitis 77
Bacteroides 250
forsythus. 102–3
bariatric surgery 293
basement membrane 67
basophils 208, 210
characteristics 209
behavioural change 274
Behçet's syndrome 68–9
Bennett movement 49
benzatropine 77
benzodiazepines
children 184–5
chronic renal failure 138–9
sedation 280
side-effects 283
beta blockers
atrial fibrillation 192
cardiovascular disease 200
heart failure 199
bile 31–2, 114–15
drugs excreted
into 117–18
pigments 114–15
salts 114–15
bilirubin 114–15
impaired liver function 128
binge eating disorder
(compulsive eating) 37
bioactive glass 96
biologic width 20
Bio-Oss® 96
bisoprolol 199

bisphosphonates 86, 104–5
bitewing dental
    radiograph 12, 102
bleeding
    chronic kidney disease 148
    chronic renal
        failure 143, 146
    disorders 222–4
    haemostasis 220–1
    history taking 130–1
    local measures to
        stop 130
    sudden blood loss,
        response to 195
    time 221
    white blood cells,
        malignancy of 227
bleomycin 185
blood
    clotting, drugs
        impairing 224
    components 208
    types 228
        clinical relevance 228
blood cancers 226–7, 246
blood cells
    characteristics 209
    formation (haemato-
        poiesis) 212–14
    functions 210–11
    types 208–11
blood glucose
    diabetes 153
    glucose tolerance test 154
    monitoring 152–5
    normal levels 153
blood pressure (BP)
    control 194
        sudden blood loss 195
    postural
        hypotension 194, 272
    see also hypertension
blood tests 221
blood transfusion 228
    doping by athletes 216–19
    leukocyte depletion 254–5
body mass index
    (BMI) 36, 158
    obesity 158
Bogorad's syndrome
    (crocodile tears) 273
Bohr shift 216–19
bone
    ageing 108–10
    anatomy 88–91
    bisphosphonates 86,
        104–5
    cells 108–10
    composition by weight 12
    diabetes 164–5
    formation 94
        mechanism 294

grafts 96, 97
    alveolar clefts 101
    healing 94–6
        extraction socket 98–9
    hormonal influences 92
    kidney transplantation
        patients 145
    matrix content 87
    metastasis 86
    mineral content 86
    orthodontic tooth
        movement 100–1
    pathology
        chronic renal
            disease 144–5
        in the elderly 106–7
    periodontal bone
        loss in chronic
            periodontitis 102–3
    remodelling 9
    resorption 12–13
        chronology 9
        clinical application 13
        control 294
        excessive 295
        inhibiting factors 13
        insufficient 295
        mechanism 294
        promoting factors 13
        severe 13
    structure 86–7
        age changes 108
        gross 88
        microscopic 88–9
    turnover 92–3
bone marrow
    blood cell
        formation 212–14
    transplantation 226–7
bone remodelling unit 92
bovine spongiform
    encephalitis (BSE) 254
brain injury 83–4
brain tumour 83–4
bronchi
    non-respiratory conducting
        system 170
    obstruction 176
bronchial carcinoma 170
bronchiectasis 170
bronchioles 170
bronchitis, chronic 180
    see also chronic obstructive
        pulmonary disease
buccal nerve 264
buffering 28
bulimia nervosa 37
bumetanide 199
bundle of His 191
bupivacaine 117, 198–9, 277
burning mouth syndrome 263
    diabetes 162–3

C

calcitonin
    bone 92, 93
    thyroid gland 298
calcium 35
calcium-channel blockers
    atrial fibrillation 192
    cardiovascular disease 200
    chronic renal failure 143
    renovascular
        hypertension 138–9
calculus 252–3
canaliculi 88
cancellous bone 88
cancer
    blood 226–7, 246
    bronchial 170
    lung 181
    neck dissection 266
    oesophageal 218
    oropharyngeal 106–7, 251
    pancreatic 151
    radiation-induced oral
        mucositis 72–3
    thyroid 301
    transplant patients 229
    white blood cells 226–7
    see also laryngeal
        cancer; oral cancer;
        pharyngeal cancer
candesartan 199
Candida 163
    albicans 251
candidiasis see oral
    candidiasis
canines
    alveolar clefts,
        management of 101
    eruption 8
    impacted, surgical
        exposure of 101
    lateral mandibular
        movements 49
Capnocytophaga 23
captopril 199
carbamazepine 56, 219, 263
carbohydrates 35
carcinogenesis 70
cardiac cycle 188, 189
cardiac failure see heart
    failure
cardiac output,
    control of 194
cardiovascular disease
    diabetes 160, 161
    general anaesthesia 184
cardiovascular implant-
    able electronic devices
    (CIED) 199
cardiovascular system,
    control of 194–5

caries 22–4
  aetiology 22
    bacterial activity 23
    free sugars 23
  asthma 181–2
  cementum 16
  chronic kidney
    disease 140–1
  diabetes 159, 162–3
  dry mouth 77, 162–3
  epidemiology 22
  infective endocarditis,
    patients at risk of 203
  prevention
    behaviour change 29
    dementia patients 285
    diet and
      nutrition 28–9, 159
    fluoride 24, 26, 27
  progression 24
  pulpal pathology 243
  risk factors and
    markers 22
carvedilol 199
cataracts 161
cellulitis 245
cellulose 35
cementoblasts 16
cementocytes 93
cementum 16, 93
  composition by weight 12
  excessive
    (hypercementosis) 16
central nervous
  system (CNS)
  disorders 272
  microglial cells 235
central pattern generator
  (CPG) 59
central sensitization 260
cerebral palsy 77
cerebrovascular accident
  (CVA) see stroke
chemokines 233
chemoreceptors 172–3
chemotaxins 243
chemotherapy
  inhalation sedation 185
  leukaemia 226–7
  lymphoma 227
  oral mucositis 72–3
  pancreatic cancer 151
cherubism 9
chewing see mastication
chewing tobacco 283
children
  asthma 182
  behaviour change 274
  benzodiazepines 184–5
  chronic renal failure 143
  diabetes 159
  drug prescribing for 283

excess fluoride
  ingestion 26
  prevention 27
herpes simplex 251
hypothyroidism
  (cretinism) 300
inhalation
  sedation 182, 184–5
leukaemia 226–7
pituitary gigantism 303
Reye's syndrome 126
chloramphenicol 219
chlorhexidine mouth rinses
  alveolar osteitis,
    prevention of 98, 99
  extraction socket 98, 99
  hypersensitivity to 246
choking 79
cholecystokinin (CCK) 32,
    292, 293
  bile 31–2
  pancreatic secretions 31
  and somatostatin 302–3
cholesterol 115
chondrocytes,
  hypertrophic 89
chorda tympani nerve 270
  taste sensation 272, 273
  trauma 273
Christmas disease
  (haemophilia B) 223
chronic obstructive pulmonary disease (COPD) 180
  anatomic dead space 175
  aspiration pneumonia 78
  comorbid GORD 177
  gas exchange 170
  heart failure 198–9
  impaired swallowing 78
  respiratory failure 171
  sedation 280
  spirometry 174, 175
chyme 30–1
chymotrypsin 150
ciclosporin
  chronic kidney
    disease 140–1, 147
  chronic renal failure 143
  transplant patients 229
cigarette smoking see
  smoking
ciliary ganglion 271
cirrhosis 122
  hepatitis B 126
cleft lip and palate
  distraction
    osteogenesis 101
  orthodontic tooth
    movement 101
  speech problems 84
  swallowing problems 79

cleidocranial dysostosis 9
clindamycin 99, 224
clopidogrel 224
clotting cascade 115
clotting studies 128
clozapine 77
coagulation
  disorders 222–3
  pathway 220
  screen 221
cocaine 282–3
codeine 281
cognitive behavioural
  therapy 50
cold sores 251
collagen 89
  diabetes 164
complement 233
  activation 237
  system 232
compulsive eating (binge
  eating disorder) 37
condylar cartilage
  lateral pterygoid
    muscle 45
  osteoarthritis 45
condylar fracture 45
condylar guidance 54
condyle 48
congestive heart failure 170
continuous positive airway
  pressure (CPAP) 179
convoluted tubule
  distal 135
  proximal 134
corbadrine 269
coronary arteries,
  atherosclerosis 196–7
coronary artery disease 179
coronary heart disease
  (CHD) 203
coronary syndrome, acute
  (ACS) 203
cortex of long bones, blood
  supply 89
cortical bone 88
  age changes 108
corticosteroids
  facial transplant 229
  hydrocortisone supple-
    mentation prior to
    surgery 297
  inhaled
    asthma 181–2, 183
    oropharyngeal
      candidiasis 181, 183
  kidney transplantation
    patients 145
corticotrophin-releasing
  hormone 296
cortisol
  Addison's disease 297

Cushing's
  syndrome 296–7
  regulation 296
cough reflex 176
cranial nerves 266–7
cretinism 300
Creutzfeldt–Jakob disease, variant (vCJD) 254–5
crevicular epithelium 19
crocodile tears (Bogorad's syndrome) 273
crown
  airway obstruction 176
  completion, chronology 9
  formation 2
cryotherapy 73
Cushing's
  syndrome 296–7
cytochrome P450
  enzymes 116–17
cytokines 233
  bone resorption, control of 294
  cell-mediated response 240
  inflammation, chronic 243
cytomegalovirus 124
cytotoxic T cells 241
  cell-mediated response 240

D

dabigatran 200, 224
darbepoetin alfa 142–3
decontamination of instruments 254
deep petrosal nerve 270
dementia 284–5
  aphasia 83–4
  aspiration pneumonia 78
  dental care 285
  denture wearing 285
  pain, recognition of 281
dendritic cells (DCs)
  cell-mediated response 240
  non-specific immune response 232
denosumab 294
dental caries see caries
dental follicle 2, 8–9
dental hard tissues, composition 12–13
  by weight 12
dental pain 260–1
dental papilla 2, 15
dental surgery see oral surgery
dental unit water lines 255
dentine 15
  caries 24, 28–9

composition by weight 12
hypersensitivity 261
pain when air-dried 260–1
types 15
dentures
  bilateral balanced occlusion 49
  dementia 285
  diabetes 163
  dry mouth 77
  inhalation of 177
  interocclusal rest space measurement 54
  jaw reflexes 56
  speech 83–4
  tardive dyskinesia 285
depression 259
desensitization, systematic 274
desmopressin
  thrombocytopenia 222
  von Willebrand's disease 223
diabetes mellitus 168
  acute symptoms 155
  Argyll–Robertson pupils 271
  atherosclerosis 196–7
  autonomic neuropathy 271
  blood glucose monitoring 152–5
  chronic kidney disease 138–9, 148
  coronary heart disease and periodontal diseases 203
  dental complications 162–3
  diagnosis 152
  epidemiology 158–9
  foot ulceration 166
  glycaemic control 156–7
  hypertension 194
  immunity, impaired 246
  infection
    poorly controlled diabetes 164–5
    severe 166–7
  insulin resistance 156–7
  liver disease 122–3
  medical complications 160–1
    macrovascular 160
    microvascular 160–1
  myocardial infarction 197
  renovascular hypertension 141
  stroke risk 204–5
  Type I diabetes 153
    dental health in children with 159

glucose tolerance test 154
  infection 166–7
  juvenile 248
  periodontitis 253
  retinopathy 160–1
Type II diabetes 153
  animal models 164
  epidemiology 158
  glucose tolerance test 154
  infection 164
  insulin resistance 156–7
  periodontal disease 162
Diabetes Risk Score assessment tool 156–7
diabetic ketoacidosis see hyperglycaemia
diabetic nephropathy 161
  chronic kidney disease 140–1
diabetic retinopathy 160–1
dialysis 140–1
  bleeding tendency 146
  oral signs and symptoms 143
  renal osteodystrophy 144
diastole 188, 189
diathermy 199
diazepam 280
diclofenac 139
diet and nutrition 34–5
  advice 34
  atherosclerosis 196–7
  caries prevention 28–9, 159
  diabetes 159, 162–3
  free sugars 28–9
  iodine deficiency 298
  iron 213
  obesity 158
  oral mucositis 73
  problems 36–7
  salivary flow 75
digastric muscle 46
digestion
  carbohydrates 35
  fat 34
  protein 34
digestive enzymes 150
digestive tract 30–3
  co-ordinating mechanisms 32
  progression along the gut 30–1
  secretions 31–2
  vomiting (emesis) 32–3
  see also diet and nutrition
digoxin 116, 192, 199
diltiazem 200
diphenhydramine 269
diplopia 279

dipyridamole 224
disseminated intravascular
    coagulation (DIC) 221
distraction osteogenesis 101
diuretics 199
    potassium-sparing 138–9
Down's syndrome 9
drug abuse 282–3
    inhalation of dentures 177
drug-induced thrombocyto-
    penic purpura 222
drugs
    anaemia 219
    cardiovascular disease 200
    chronic renal
        failure 138–9
    common interactions 283
    heart failure 199
    interactions 117
    metabolism 116–17, 131
    prescribing for
        children 283
dry mouth
    causes 76
    diabetes 162–3
    lung disease 181–2
    management 77
    problems arising from 77
'dry socket' see alveolar
    osteitis
Duchenne muscular
    dystrophy 62
dysaesthesia 262
dysarthria 82
dyskinesia 284–5
    denture wearing 285
dysphagia 78–9
    stroke patients 204
dysphasia see aphasia
dystonia 284

E

early bruising
    syndrome 222–4
eating disorders 36–7
ecstasy (MDMA) 282
ectoderm 2
ectomesenchyme 2
edentulous patients
    interocclusal rest space
        measurement 54
    jaw muscle activity and
        composition 61
    see also dentures
Ehlers–Danlos syndrome 87
Eikonella 250
elderly patients
    bone pathology 106–7
    plasma protein binding of
        drugs 116
    sedation 280

electric pulp tester 199
electrocardiogram
    (ECG) 191–2
    cardiac cycle 189
    normal 191
electrosurgery 199
elevator muscles 40–1
    fibres 60–1
    hyperactivity, clinical
        significance of 41–2
embryonic development 2
emesis see vomiting
emphysema 180
    see also chronic obstructive
        pulmonary disease
enamel 14
    asthma 182
    caries 24, 28–9
    composition by weight 12
    hypoplasia 143
    maturation 6
    prisms 14
    surface 14
enamel organ 2, 14
endochondral
    ossification 94, 95–6
endoderm 2
endodontic disease 162
endorphins 261
endothelial erosion/
    dysfunction 196–7
enophthalmos 271
entecavir 140–1
enterokinase 150
eosinophils 208, 210
    characteristics 209
    inflammation, chronic 243
epidermal growth factor
    receptor (EGFR) 70
epinephrine see adrenaline
eplerenone 199
eptifibatide 224
Epworth sleepiness
    score 178–9
erythrocytes see red
    blood cells
erythromycin
    avoidance in patients
        with impaired liver
        function 131
    drug interactions 200,
        224, 283
erythroplakia 71
erythropoietin 136–7,
    142–3, 148
    doping by athletes 216–19
    recombinant 146
ethnicity, and stroke
    risk 204–5
Eubacterium 23
exenatide 293
exfoliation, chronology 9

expressive aphasia 83–4
extraction, tooth 276
extraction socket
    diabetes 164, 167
    healing of the 98–9, 164
    medication-related
        osteonecrosis of the
        jaw (MRONJ) 104–5
eye movement, lesions of
    nerves causing 267

F

face masks 255–6
facial artery
    mandible 91
    maxillary bone 91
facial nerve (cranial nerve
    VII) 266, 270
    digastric muscle 40–2, 46
    palsy 278
    speech production 82–4
    taste sensation 272, 273
    trauma 273
facial pain 260–1
facial skin sensation 264–5
facial transplant 229
factor VIII therapy 223
factor IX therapy 223
fainting (syncope) 194–5
fats, dietary 34
feedback, for behaviour
    change 274
fentanyl 281
ferritin 213
fibre, dietary 35
fibrinogen assay 221
fixed orthodontic
    treatment 100
fluconazole 131, 200
flumazenil 184–5, 280
fluorapatite (FAP) 26
fluoride
    asthma 182
    bone 86
    caries prevention 24, 26, 27
    dementia patients 285
    diabetes 162–3
    eating disorders 37
    excess 26–7
    metabolism 27
    mouth rinse 37
fluorosis 26, 27
follicle stimulating
    hormone (FSH)
    men 290
    women 288–90
    menstrual cycle 288–9
follicular carcinoma 301
foot ulceration, diabetic 166
forced expiratory volume in
    1 s (FEV1) 174, 175

lung disease 174
forced vital capacity
(FVC) 174, 175
lung disease 174
foreign object, inhalation of
dentures 177
gas exchange 170
fracture
condylar 45
long bones 94, 95
maturation of newly
calcified tissue 95–6
matrix 94
free sugars 23
caries prevention 28–9
Stephan curve 28–9
freeway space 54
fresh frozen plasma 130–1
Frey's syndrome 273
functional residual capacity
(FRC) 174, 175
fungi, oral 251
furosemide 199
Fusobacteria 23, 250

G

gamma-glutamyl transferase
(GGT) 128
ganglionic branch, trigeminal
nerve 265
Gardner's syndrome 9
gastric motility 30–1
gastric secretions 31
gastrin 32, 292
and somatostatin 302–3
gastrointestinal
hormones 292–3
gastro-oesophageal reflux
disease (GORD) 177
gender factors
anaemia 216–19
atherosclerosis 196–7
drug metabolism in the
liver 117
haemophilia A 223
haemophilia B 223
myocardial infarction 197
obesity 158
general anaesthesia
(GA) 184
avoidance in patients
with impaired liver
function 131
heart failure 198–9
infective endocarditis,
patients at risk of 203
inhalation of dentures,
prevention of 177
mechanism of action 280–1
sickle cell disorder
screening 219

thalassaemia
screening 219
geniohyoid muscle 47
ghrelin 150–1, 292, 293
gigantism, pituitary 303
gingival crevicular fluid
(GCF) 20
gingival fibre groups 19
gingival fibromatosis,
hereditary 9
gingivitis 102–3
asthma 183
glaucoma 161
glomerular filtration
rate 136–7
glomerulonephritis 247
glossopharyngeal nerve
(cranial nerve IX)
266, 270
taste sensation 272, 273
glucagon 150–1
and somatostatin 302–3
glucagon-like peptide-1
(GLP-1) 293
glucocorticoids
kidney transplantation
patients 145
transplant patients 229
gluconeogenesis 150–1
central obesity 158
glucose
blood see blood glucose
intolerance 153
resistance 156
glucose-dependent insuli-
notropic polypeptide
(GIP) 293
glucose tolerance
test 154
glycaemic control 156–7
glycated haemoglobin
(HbA1c) 152
diabetic diagnosis 152
diabetic retinopathy 160–1
insulin resistance 157
glycation end products 152
glyceryl trinitrate (GTN)
angina 196–7
myocardial infarction 197
prophylactic 197
glycopyrronium bromide 77
goitre 299, 300
multinodular
(MNG) 300, 301
Golgi tendon organ reflexes
and muscle spindle
reflexes, difference
between 58
physiology 58
gonadotrophin-releasing
hormone (GnRH)
men 290

women 288–90
menstrual cycle 288
granuloma 243
Graves' disease 300
goitre 300
great auricular nerve 264
greater petrosal
nerve 272
growth factors 165
growth hormone 302–3
abnormalities 303
actions 303
regulation 302
growth hormone releasing
hormone (GHRH)
growth hormone
regulation 302–3
pituitary gigantism 303
guided tissue
regeneration 103
Guillain–Barré
syndrome 271
gustatory sweating 273
gut see digestive tract

H

haemodialysis see dialysis
haemoglobin
anaemia 216–19
sickle cell 218–19
dissociation curve 216
haemolytic anaemia 247
haemolytic disease of the
newborn 228
haemophilia A 223
haemophilia B (Christmas
disease) 223
Haemophilus 250
haemorrhagic disease of
newborn 223–4
haemosiderin 213
haemostasis 220–1
bleeding disorders 222–4
haemotopoiesis 212–14
haemotopoietic stem cells
(HSC) 212–14
haloperidol 269
halothane 281
hard tissues see dental hard
tissues, composition
Hashimoto's disease 301
goitre 300
hay fever 246
heart
arrhythmias 192
contraction, control
of 190–2
function 188–9
infections 202–3
transplantation 199
valves 189

heart block 192
heart failure 198–9
  atrial fibrillation 192
  clinical presentation 198
  clinical relevance 198–9
  drug metabolism in the liver 117
  management 198, 199
Henoch Schönlein purpura 222–4
heparin 221, 224
hepatic encephalopathy 123
hepatitis 124–6
  A 124
  alcoholic 122
  B 124–6
    blood tests 126
    chronic kidney disease 140–1
    immunization 256
    inoculation injuries 256
    prevention 126
    serological markers 125
    symptoms 124–6
    treatment 126
    vaccine 238
  C 124
    chronic kidney disease 140–1
    injecting drug users 282
    inoculation injuries 256
  D 124
  E 124
  paracetamol overdose 117
  types 124
hepato-renal syndrome 131
herd immunity 238
hereditary haemorrhagic telangiectasia 222–4
Hering-Breuer reflex 173
heroin 282–3
herpes labialis lesions 251
herpes simplex 251
histamine 233
HIV/AIDS 246
  injecting drug users 282
  inoculation injuries 256
  post-exposure prophylaxis 256
  T helper cells 240
Hodgkin lymphoma 227
Horner's syndrome 271
Howship's lacunae 92, 294
human leukocyte antigen (HLA) 229
human papilloma virus (HPV) 251
  oral cancer 106–7
humoral response 235–6
hunger centre, hypothalamus 34–5

hyalinization zone, orthodontic tooth movement 100
hydrodynamic hypothesis 260–1
hydroxyapatite (HAP) 26
  grafts 96
1,25 hydroxyvitamin D$_3$ 294
hyoscine hydrobromide 77
hyperbaric oxygen
  diabetic foot ulceration 166
  medication-related osteonecrosis of the jaw (MRONJ) 104–5
hypercementosis 16
hyperglycaemia
  diabetes 151, 155
  dry mouth 162–3
  infection 166–7
  glycation end products 152
  post-prandial 153
  stress response 164
hyperinsulinaemia 158
hyperkeratinization 66
hyperparathyroidism
  bone resorption 295
  chronic kidney disease 144, 145
  vitamin D 93
hypersensitivity 246–7
hypertension 194
  atherosclerosis 196–7
  atrial fibrillation 192
  chronic kidney disease 138–9, 148
  coronary heart disease and periodontal diseases 203
  diabetic retinopathy 160–1
  essential 194
  heart failure 198–9
  obstructive sleep apnoea 178–9
  portal see portal hypertension
  renovascular 138–9, 140–1
  stroke
    prevention 160
    risk 204–5
hyperthyroidism 299, 300
  atrial fibrillation 192
  clinical features 300
hypertrophic chondrocytes 89
hyperventilation 171
hypoglossal nerve (cranial nerve XII) 266
hypoglycaemia
  diabetes 155
    infection 166–7
    treatment 168
  pancreas 150–1

hyposalivation, drug-induced 76
hypotension, postural 194, 272
hypothyroidism 298, 299, 300
  clinical features 300
  delayed tooth eruption 9
hypoxia inducible factor-1 (HIF-1) 142–3

I

ibuprofen 139, 281
ice chips 73
imipramine 269
immune complex reaction, type III 222–4
immune system
  cell-mediated response 240
  dental plaque 252–3
  inflammation 242–5
  mediators 232, 233
  non-specific defences 232
  oral flora 250–1
  problems 246–8
  specific defences 234–7
immune thrombocytopenic purpura 222
immune tolerance 234
immunization 238
immunodeficiency
  congenital 246
  diseases 246
immunoglobulins (Ig) 115
  IgA 236–7
  IgD 237
  IgE 237
    hypersensitivity 246, 247
  IgG 236–7
    hypersensitivity 247
    immunization 238
  IgM 236–7
    hypersensitivity 247
    immunization 238
  structure 236
immunosuppression 229, 246
  adverse effects 229
  autoimmune disease 248
impacted canines, surgical exposure of 101
impacted third molars
  extraction 98–9
  risk factors 263
implants 164
impression taking, retching during 33
incisal (anterior) guidance 54–5

incisive nerve 264
indometacin 139
infection
  control 254–6
  dental 243
    spread to tissue
      spaces 245
infective endocarditis
  (IE) 202
  clinical relevance 203
inferior alveolar artery 91
inferior alveolar nerve 264
  block
    complications 278–9
    procedure 278
  damage to, as com-
    plication of local
    anaesthesia 278
inflammation 242–5
  acute 242
  aftermath 243–5
  chronic 243
  dental 243
  gingival 252
  mediators 232, 233, 242
  periodontal 252–3
infrahyoid muscles 46
  temporomandibular
    joint 48
infraorbital nerve 265
inhalation of foreign object
  see foreign object,
    inhalation of
inhalation sedation see
  sedation: inhalation
inhibin
  men 290
  women 289
inoculation injuries 256
instrument
  decontamination 254
insulin 150–1
  Cushing's syndrome 296–7
  diabetes 164
  resistance 153, 154,
    156–7
    central obesity 158
    continuous positive
      airway pressure 179
    obstructive sleep
      apnoea 178–9
    periodontal disease 162
  and somatostatin 302–3
insulin-like growth factor
  actions 303
  growth hormone
    regulation 302–3
insulinomas 151
interferons 233
  hepatitis B 126
interleukins (IL) 233
  IL-1 235

internal maxillary artery 91
international normalized
  ratio (INR) 221, 224
  impaired liver
    function 128
interocclusal rest space 54
intrafusal fibres 58–9
intramembranous
  ossification 94, 95–6
intravenous induction
  agents 138–9
intrinsic factor 31
invasive external
  otitis 166–7
iodine deficiency 298, 300
  goitre 300
iron 35
  deficiency
    oral mucosa, effect
      on 71–2
    see also anaemia
  metabolism 213
ischaemic heart
  disease 198–9
islets of Langerhans 150–1
  tumours 151
isoflurane
  clinical relevance 281
  mechanism of
    action 280–1
isosorbide
  mononitrate 199

jaundice 114–15
  dental care in patients
    with 130
  drug metabolism 131
  pancreatic cancer 151
jaw
  age changes 108
  blood supply 91
  bone grafts 96
  mandibular advancement
    prostheses 179
  mandibular side shift 49
  medication-related
    osteonecrosis of the
    (MRONJ) 104–5
  movements 48–9
    clinical
      considerations 54–5
    extreme border
      movements 55
  muscles see muscles: of
    mastication
  osteomyelitis 167
jaw jerk reflex 56
  clinical significance 57
  exaggerated 56
jaw opening reflex 19

jaw reflexes 56–7
junctional epithelium 19–20

K
kanamycin 139
Kawasaki disease (KD) 69
keratinocyte growth
  factor 73
ketoacidosis 166–7
kidney disease, chronic
  (CKD) 140–1, 148
  anaemia 142–3
  bone pathology 144–5
  classification 138–9
  drug metabolism 117, 138
  hypertension 194
  mineral and bone disorder
    (CKD-MBD) 144
  stages 139
kidneys
  anatomy 134–5
  failure see renal failure,
    chronic
  functions 136–7
    bicarbonate
      reabsorption,
      regulation of 136
    filtration
      mechanism 136
    sodium and chloride
      ion balance,
      regulation of 137
  structure 136–7
  transplantation 145
  see also kidney disease,
    chronic
kinins 233
Kupffer cells 235

L
lachrymal nerve 270
lachrymation 270
lactobacilli 23, 250
lactose 23
lactulose 123
lamellar bone 89, 90, 98–9
lamina propria 67
large intestine 30–1
laryngeal cancer
  airway obstruction 176
  dysphagia 78–9
  laser treatment 73
laser treatment 73
lateral mandibular
  movements 49
  clinical significance 49
lateral pterygoid
  muscle 44–5
  clinical significance 44–5
  temporomandibular
    joint 48–9

latex,
    hypersensitivity to 246
Le Fort I osteotomy maxil-
    lary segment 91
learning disability 77
lecithin 115
Legionella 255
leptin 150–1
lesser petrosal nerve 270
leucocytes see white
    blood cells
leukaemia 226–7
leukoplakia 70
levodopa-induced
    dyskinesia 285
lichen planus 248
lidocaine (lignocaine)
    applications 276
    chronic renal failure 139
    comparison with other
        local anaesthetics 277
    metabolism in the liver 117
    mode of action 276
    properties 276–7
lingual artery 91
lingual nerve
    damage 262, 273
    local anaesthesia 278
    taste sensation 272, 273
lipase 150
lisinopril 200
liver
    anatomy 112–13
    chronic kidney
        disease 140–1
    drugs 116–18
    function tests 128
    functions 114–15
        exocrine 114–15
        impaired see impaired
            function below
        metabolism of nutrients
            and toxins 114
        synthesis 115
    hepatitis see hepatitis
    impaired function
        dental care in patients
            with 130–1
        drugs to avoid 131
    Kupffer cells 235
    structure 112
    transplantation 126
liver disease 122–3
    bleeding disorders 223
    drug metabolism 117
liver failure
    alcohol 122
    key signs 123
    plasma protein binding of
        drugs 116
local anaesthesia
    (LA) 276–7

avoidance in patients
    with impaired liver
    function 131
biotransformation of
    epinephrine in 269
bleeding disorders 224
cardiovascular disease 200
chronic kidney
    disease 148
chronic renal failure 139
clinical relevance 276
comparison 277
dental 278–9
drug interactions 283
heart failure 198–9
    implanted devices 199
maxillary infiltration 276–7
metabolism in the
    liver 117
mode of action 276
overdose 276
properties 276–7
side-effects 276
stroke patients 204
localized airway
    obstruction 176–7
long bones
    cortex, blood supply 89
    fracture healing 94, 95
    maturation of newly
        calcified tissue 95–6
long buccal nerve 264
loop of Henle
    analgesic
        nephropathy 138–9
    ascending 134, 137
    descending 134
lorazepam 280
losartan 199
lung cancer 181
lung disease 180–3
    FEV1 and FVC 174
    general anaesthesia 184
    see also asthma; chronic
        obstructive pulmonary
        disease; lung cancer
lungs
    structure and
        function 170–1
    volume changes during
        respiration 174
luteinizing hormone (LH)
    men 290
    women 288–90
    menstrual cycle 288–9
lymphoblastic leukaemia,
    acute (ALL) 226–7
lymphocytes 208, 210
    characteristics 209
    inflammation, chronic 243
    specific immune
        response 235

see also B lymphocytes;
    T lymphocytes
lymphocytic leukaemia,
    chronic 226–7
lymphokines 240
lymphoma 227

M

macrophages 210, 235
    cell-mediated response 240
    inflammation, chronic 243
    non-specific immune
        response 232
    platelet destruction 213
    red blood cell
        destruction 212
magnetic resonance imaging
    (MRI) 199
major histocompatibility
    complex (MHC) 234
    cell-mediated response 240
malnutrition 116
mandible see jaw
mandibular advancement
    prostheses 179
mandibular side shift 49
masseter muscle 40
    composition variation
        between species 61
    temporomandibular
        joint 48, 49
mast cells 210
    non-specific immune
        response 232
mastication
    anterior guidance 54–5
    central pattern
        generator 59
    crocodile tears (Bogorad's
        syndrome) 273
    dry mouth 77
    muscles of see muscles: of
        mastication
    occlusion 52
    periodontal receptors 57
masticatory–salivary
    reflex 19
matrix metalloproteinases
    (MMPs) 180
maxilla
    bisphosphonate-induced
        osteonecrosis 104–5
    blood supply 91
maxillofacial injury 176
maximal intercuspal position
    (MIP) 54
MDMA (methylenedioxym-
    ethamphetamine) 282
mean arterial pressure
    (MAP) 194
mechanoreceptors (gut) 32

medial pterygoid
  muscle 41, 42
  temporomandibular
    joint 48–9
median rhomboid
  glossitis 163
medication-related
  osteonecrosis of the
  jaw (MRONJ) 104–5
medullary respiratory
  pattern generator 173
medullary thyroid
  carcinoma 301
memory cells 210,
  235, 241
  immunization 238
menopause 106, 108, 295
menstrual cycle 288–9
mental nerve 264
mepivacaine 117, 277
mesencephalic nucleus,
  trigeminal nerve 53
  jaw jerk reflex 56
  unloading reflex 56
mesenchymal stem
  cells (MSC)
  age changes 108, 109–10
  fracture healing 95
mesoderm 2
methylenedioxy-
  methamphetamine
  (MDMA) 282
meticillin-resistant
  Staphylococcus aureus
  (MRSA) 166–7
metronidazole
  alveolar osteitis,
    prevention of 99
  avoidance in patients
    with impaired liver
    function 131
  chronic kidney
    disease 138–9
  drug
    interactions 224, 283
miconazole 131, 200, 283
microglial cells 235
midazolam 117, 280
middle superior alveolar
  nerve 265
migraine 263
minerals 35
modelling 274
monocyte–macrophage
  system 210
monocytes 208, 210
  characteristics 209
motor nucleus, trigeminal
  nerve 53
motor reflexes
  jaw 56–7
  physiology of 58–9

mouth breathing
  asthma 183
  chronic obstructive pulmo-
    nary disease 181
mouth cancer see oral cancer
mouth rinse
  antiseptic see antiseptic
    mouth rinses
  fluoride 37
  mucositis 73
muco-periosteum 66
mucositis, radiation-induced
  oral 72–3
multinodular goitre
  (MNG) 300, 301
multiple myeloma 226–7
  bisphosphonates 86
multiple sclerosis (MS) 263
  aspiration pneumonia 78
  jaw jerk reflex 57
  trigeminal neuralgia
    symptoms 56
multiple system atrophy
  (MSA) 272
muscle fibres 60–1
  characteristics 60
muscle spindles
  afferent innervation 59
  efferent innervation 59
  reflexes
    clinical significance 59
    and Golgi tendon organ
      reflexes, difference
      between 58
    physiology 58
muscles
  diseases 62–3
  function 62
    and nerve func-
      tion, relationship
      between 60–1
  growth hormone 303
  hypertrophy 63
  of mastication 40–7
    activity and
      composition 61
    elevator muscle
      hyperactivity, clinical
      significance of 41–2
  neuromuscular
    junction 60–1
  physiology 56–7
  regeneration following
    injury 63
  reinnervation 61
  structure 61
Mycobacterium 255
  tuberculosis 183
mycophenolate mofetil 229
myeloid leukaemia
  acute (AML) 226–7
  chronic (CML) 226–7

mylohyoid muscle 47
myocardial infarction
  (MI) 197
  arrhythmias
    following 192
  atrial fibrillation 192
  clinical relevance 197
  heart failure 198–9
  oral bacteria 203
myocardial
  ischaemia 196–7
myofibrils 61
myotonic dystrophy 62
myxoedema 298

N

naïve T
  lymphocytes 235, 241
naproxen 139
natural killer (NK) cells 234
nausea
  dialysis 143
  inhalation sedation 185
neck dissection 266
necrotizing sialometaplasia
  (NS) 69
Neisseria 250
neomycin 123, 139
nephropathy see diabetic
  nephropathy
nerve conduction 258–9
nerve function and muscle
  function, relationship
  between 60–1
neural crest cells 2, 15
neurodegenerative
  conditions
  aspiration pneumonia 78
  bronchial obstruction 176
  neurological disease 83–4
neuromuscular
  junction 40, 62
neuropeptides 233
  neuropeptide Y 292
neurotransmitters 261
neutropenia 246
neutrophils 208, 210
  characteristics 209
nickel allergy 247
nicotine replacement
  therapy 181
nifedipine 200
nitric oxide 233
nitrous
  oxide 116–17, 184–5
  actions 185
  side-effects 283
non-Hodgkin
  lymphoma 227
non-respiratory conducting
  system 170

non-steroidal anti-inflammatory drugs (NSAIDs)
anaemia 219
analgesia 281
avoidance in patients with impaired liver function 130, 131
chronic renal failure 138, 139
contraindicated in bleeding disorders 224
side-effects 281
and warfarin, interaction between 200
non-working side of the mandible 49
occlusal interference 52
norepinephrine (noradrenaline) 268–73
novel oral anticoagulants (NOACs) 200
nuclear bag fibres 58
nuclear chain fibres 59
nursing homes, and dentures 285
nutrition see diet and nutrition

O
OAB antigens and antibodies 228, 229
obesity 36
bariatric surgery 293
central 158
coronary heart disease and periodontal diseases 203
defining 158
diabetes 153
complications 160–1
epidemiology 158
periodontal disease 162
gastrointestinal hormones 292–3
insulin resistance 156–7
liver disease 122–3
obstructive sleep apnoea 178–9
peptide tyrosine tyrosine 292
risks associated with 158, 204–5
obstructive sleep apnoea (OSA) 178–9
occlusion 52–3
anterior (incisal) guidance 54–5
bilateral balanced 49
chewing 52
clinical considerations 54–5

condylar guidance 54
elevator muscle hyperactivity 41–2
interocclusal rest space (freeway space) 54
mandibular advancement prostheses 179
maximal intercuspal position (MIP) 54
mutually protected 52
non-working side contacts 52
rest position 54
trigeminal nuclei 53
oculomotor nerve 270
eye movement 267
odontoblast process 15
odontoblasts
dentine formation 15
pain 260–1
oesophageal cancer 218
oesophagus 30–1
obstruction 77
oestrogen 288–90
menstrual cycle 288–9
olfactory nerve (cranial nerve I) 266
oncogenes 70
oncogenesis 70
opioids
analgesia 281
overdose 281
optic nerve (cranial nerve II) 266
oral cancer 70–3
age factors 106–7
alcohol 282
bone invasion 106
bone resorption 106–7
development 70
diagnosis 72
dysphagia 78–9
erythroplakia 71
human papilloma virus 251
leukoplakia 70
management 72
mandible 91
potentially malignant lesions 70
risk factors 106–7
screening 73
smoking 283
spread 72
oral candidiasis
asthma 181–2
diabetes 162–3
dry mouth 77
inhaled corticosteroids 181–2
oral cavity 2–29
oral contraception 99
oral dysaesthesia 162–3

oral epithelial dysplasia 71
oral flora 250–1
oral hygiene
asthma 183
behavioural change 274, 275
chronic kidney disease 147
dementia patients and their carers 285
heart transplant patients 199
infective endocarditis, patients at risk of 203
medication-related osteonecrosis of the jaw (MRONJ), prevention 104
mucositis 73
planned behaviour, theory of 274
self-efficacy 275
stroke patients 204
swallowing problems 78
oral mucosa
effects of iron deficiency, alcohol, and smoking 71–2
layers 66
normal structure and function 66, 67
oral mucositis, radiation-induced 72–3
oral surgery
chronic renal failure 146
diabetes 164
antibiotic prophylaxis 168
oral ulceration 68–9
oropharyngeal cancer 106–7, 251
orthodontic tooth movement 100–1, 295
osseointegration 96
osteoarthritis
lateral pterygoid muscle 45
stabilization splint therapy 51
osteoblasts 88–9
age changes 109–10
bone formation mechanism 294
bone remodelling unit 92
bone resorption mechanism 294
diabetes 164
orthodontic tooth movement 295
osteoclasts 12–13, 88–9
age changes 109
bisphosphonates 104–5

bone formation
  mechanism 294
bone remodelling unit 92
bone resorption
  control 294
  insufficient 295
  mechanism 294
  oral cancer 106–7
  periodontitis,
    chronic 102–3
osteocytes 88
  age changes 108
  bone remodelling unit 92
  orthodontic tooth
    movement 295
osteogenesis imperfecta
  bisphosphonates 86
  bone structure 87
osteomalacia
  chronic kidney
    disease 144, 145
  vitamin D 93
osteomyelitis 295
  jaw 167
osteopetrosis 295
  medication-related
    osteonecrosis of the
    jaw (MRONJ) 104–5
osteoporosis
  bisphosphonates 86,104–5
  bone structure 87
  fluoride treatment 86
  kidney transplantation
    patients 145
  mandibular cortex, thinning
    of the 108
  post-menopausal 106, 295
  RANKL and OPG 92
osteoprotegerin (OPG) 92
  bone resorption,
    control of 294
  cementocytes 93
  oral cancer 106–7
  periodontitis, chronic 102–3
osteoradionecrosis 91
otitis, invasive
  external 166–7
overweight 36
oxyntomodulin 293
ozone therapy 104–5

P

pacemakers 199
Paget's disease 86, 104–5
pain
  anatomical pathways 260
  central processing of
    painful stimuli 260
  chronic 262–3
  dental 260–1
  facial 260–1

history taking 281
inferior alveolar nerve
  block 279
modifying patient
  behaviour 274–5
neurotransmitters 261
perception 261, 262–3
referred 265, 269
see also analgesia
palatal suture, orthodontic
  tooth movement 100
Palifermin® 73
pancreas
  anatomy 150–1
  functions 150–1
pancreatic cancer 151
pancreatic
  polypeptide 150–1, 293
pancreatic secretions 31
panic attack 171
papillary thyroid carcinoma
  (PTC) 301
paracetamol
  (acetaminophen)
  analgesia 281
  asthma 182
  avoidance in patients
    with impaired liver
    function 131
  chronic kidney
    disease 138–9
  chronic renal failure 139
  metabolism in the
    liver 117
  overdose 117
paraesthesia 262
parasympathetic nervous
  system 268–73
  ganglion and effector
    receptors 268
parathyroid glands 298
parathyroid hormone
  (PTH) 294
  bone 92, 93
  chronic kidney disease 144
  normal response 144
  primary hyperparathy-
    roidism 295
Parkinson's
  disease 259, 272
  aspiration pneumonia 78
  excess saliva 77
  levodopa-induced
    dyskinesia 285
parotid salivary gland 74
  control of secretion 75
parotid sialosis 122
Paterson–Brown–Kelly
  syndrome 218
pathogen associated
  molecular pattern
  (PAMP) 232

patient behaviour,
  modifying 274–5
pattern recognition
  receptors (PRRs) 232
pemphigoid 248
pemphigus vulgaris 248
penicillin 139
peptide tyrosine tyrosine
  (PYY) 292, 293
peri-implantitis 162
periodontal bone
  loss in chronic
    periodontitis 102–3
  assessment 102
  epidemiology 102
  morphology 103
periodontal disease
  diabetes 162
  infective endocarditis,
    patients at risk of 203
  RANKL 294
  smoking 283
periodontal fibre groups 18
periodontal ligament 18–20
  Sharpey's fibres 16
  tooth eruption 8, 9
periodontal receptors 57
periodontal tissues 18–20
periodontitis 243
  chronic
    classification 103
    periodontal bone loss see
      periodontal bone loss
      in chronic periodontitis
  chronic obstructive pulmo-
    nary disease 181
  coronary heart
    disease 203
  and systemic disease 253
peripheral autonomic
  neuropathy 271
peripheral sensitization 260
peristalsis 30–1
permanent teeth
  chronology of
    development 9, 11
  eruption dates 10
pernicious anaemia 248
personal protective
  equipment (PPE) 255–6
pharyngeal artery 91
pharyngeal cancer
  dysphagia 78–9
  Plummer–Vinson
    syndrome 218
pharyngeal obstruction 77
phenindione 200, 224
phenytoin 116, 219
phobias 274
phonation 82–4
physiological dead
  space 171

318   INDEX

pilocarpine 77
pituitary gigantism 303
planned behaviour,
    theory of 274
plaque
  bacterial activity 23
  body's response 252–3
  formation 23
  periodontitis,
      chronic 102–3
  see also caries
plasma 208
  transfusion 228
plasma albumin 115, 116
plasma cells 243
plasma proteins 116, 131
platelet activating factor
    (PAF) 233
platelets 208, 211
  characteristics 209
  defects 222
  formation 213
  haemostasis 220–1
plexus of Raschkow 15, 261
Plummer–Vinson syndrome
    (PVS) 218
pneumonia
  aspiration see aspiration
      pneumonia
  as complication of inhaled
      foreign object 177
  gas exchange 170
pneumotaxic centre 173
poliomyelitis 63
polycythaemia 219
Porphyromonas
  gingivalis 102–3, 203
portal hypertension 122
  hepatic
      encephalopathy 123
posterior superior alveolar
    nerve 265
post-menopausal
    osteoporosis 106
postural
  hypotension 194, 272
posture, maintenance of 58
potassium-sparing
    diuretics 138–9
potassium
  supplements 138–9
prasugrel 224
precementum
  pregnancy 16
alcohol
    recommendations 120
calcitonin 93
goitre 300
plasma proteins 116
premolars, eruption 8
pressure zone, orthodontic
    tooth movement 100

prilocaine
  comparison with other
      local anaesthetics 277
  metabolism in the
      liver 117
  mode of action 276
  properties 276–7
primary teeth
  chronology of
      development 9, 11
  eruption 9
  dates 10
prions 254
progesterone 289
  menstrual cycle 288–9
Propionibacterium 23
propofol 117, 138–9, 280–1
propranolol 122, 200
prostaglandins (PGs) 233
proteases 150
protein 34
prothrombin time (PT) 221
  coagulation screen 221
  impaired liver function 128
proton pump inhibitor (PPI)
    therapy 177
Pseudomonas 250
  aeruginosa 166–7
  dental unit water
      lines 255
pterygoid muscle see lateral
    pterygoid muscle; medial
    pterygoid muscle
pterygoid venous plexus,
    haematoma in the 279
ptosis 271
pulmonary artery and
    vein 172
pulmonary oedema 170
pulp–dentine complex 15
pulp necrosis 243
pulpal pathology 243
pulpitis 243
  local anaesthesia 276
Purkinje fibres 191
purpura 222–4
pus 244

Q
quorum sensing 250–1

R
radiation-induced oral
    mucositis 72–3
radiotherapy
  dry mouth 76
  leukaemia 226–7
  lymphoma 227
  multiple myeloma 226–7
  oral mucositis 72–3

osteoradionecrosis 91
pancreatic cancer 151
ramipril 141, 199, 200
RANK ligand (RANKL) 92
  age changes 109
  bone resorption,
      control of 294
  cementocytes 93
  kidney transplantation
      patients 145
  oral cancer 106–7
  orthodontic tooth
      movement 295
  periodontitis,
      chronic 102–3
receptive aphasia 83–4
receptor activator of
    nuclear factor kappa-B
    ligand (RANKL) see
    RANK ligand
rectum 31
recurrent aphthous
    stomatitis (RAS) 68–9
red blood cells (RBCs,
    erythrocytes) 208, 211
  anaemia 216–19
  characteristics 209
  formation 142, 143, 212
  iron metabolism 213
  types 228
Reed–Sternberg cells 227
referred pain 265, 269
renal disease, chronic see
    kidney disease, chronic
renal failure, chronic (CRF)
  anaemia 142–3, 146
  bleeding
      tendency 143, 146
  dialysis patients, oral signs
      and symptoms 143
  drug prescription 138–9
  jaundice 131
  plasma protein binding of
      drugs 116
renal function 134–5
renal osteodystrophy 144
renin 135
renin–angiotensin–
    aldosterone system 137,
    140–1
  heart failure 198–9
  sudden blood loss,
      response to 195
renovascular hyperten-
    sion 138–9, 140–1
reproductive
  hormones 288–90
  female 288–90
  male 290
residual volume 174, 175
resorption see under bone
respiratory drive 171

respiratory failure
  type 1: 171
  type 2: 171
respiratory system
  anaesthesia and
    sedation 184–5
  control of respiratory
    exchange 172–3
  localized airway
    obstruction 176–7
  lung disease 180–3
  lung structure and
    function 170–1
  obstructive sleep
    apnoea 178–9
  physiology 174–5
resting potential 258
resuscitation 176
retching 32–3
  clinical relevance 33
retinopathy, diabetic 160–1
Reye's syndrome 126, 283
Rhesus antigens 228
  hypersensitivity 247
rheumatic fever 202
rheumatoid arthritis 248
rhinocerebral
  mucormycosis 166–7
rhomboid glossitis,
  median 163
rickets 9
rivaroxaban 200, 224
root caries 24
root completion 9
root formation 2, 6
  tooth eruption 8–9
root resorption 100

S

salbutamol 182
saliva 74–7
  autonomic nervous
    system 270
  constituents 74
    with flow 75, 76
  dry mouth, causes of 76
  excess 77
  flow
    and composition 28
    problems,
      investigation 77
  functions 74
  hypersecretion 77
  production 75
    reduced see dry mouth
  secretion 74
    control 75
  Sjögren's syndrome 76
salivary glands 74
  biopsy 77
  control of secretion 75

satiety centre,
  hypothalamus 34–5
scalers see ultrasonic scalers
scurvy 87, 222–4
secretin 32, 292
  and somatostatin 302–3
sedation 184–5
  avoidance in patients
    with impaired liver
    function 131
  drugs 280
  heart failure 198–9
  inhalation 184–5
    asthma 182
    contraindications 185
    technique 185
    side-effects 283
Selenomonas 250
self-efficacy 275
senile purpura 222–4
sensory nucleus, trigeminal
  nerve 53
serotonin 233
serum 208
  bilirubin 128
sevoflurane 280–1
Sharpey's fibres 16
sharps injuries 256
shock 117
sialadenitis, bacterial 77
sialography 77
sialometry 77
sialorrhoea 77
sialosis 122
sickle cell anaemia 218–19
  screening 219
sickle cell trait 219
silent period 56–7
  clinical significance 57
simvastatin 200
sinoatrial (SA) node 190–2
  arrhythmias 192
Sjögren's syndrome 76
skeletal hormones 294–5
small intestine 30–1
smoking 283
  alveolar osteitis 99
  asthma 183
  atherosclerosis 196–7
  COPD 177, 180, 181
  coronary heart disease
    and periodontal
    diseases 203
  GORD 177
  obstructive sleep
    apnoea 178–9
  oral cancer 106–7
  oral mucosa, effect
    on 71–2
stroke
  prevention 160
  risk 204–5

somatostatin 150–1, 292
  growth hormone
    regulation 302–3
sotalol 200
speech 82–4
  dental procedures, effects
    on 83–4
  dry mouth 77
  problems 76, 82
    clinical application
      83–4
  production 82–4
spermatogenesis 290
spinal tract nucleus,
  trigeminal nerve 53
spindles see muscle spindles
spirometry 174, 175
spironolactone 199
splatter 255
  fate 255
  infection control 255
splenic macrophages 235
splints see anterior repositioning splint; stabilization
  splint therapy
squamous cell
  carcinoma 266
stabilization splint
  therapy 50, 51
staff protection 255–6
Staphylococcus aureus
  meticillin-resistant 166–7
  osteomyelitis 167
Starling's law of the
  heart 194
statins 200
stem cell transplantation
  leukaemia 226–7
  multiple myeloma 226–7
  osteopetrosis 295
Stephan curve 28
sterilization of
  instruments 254
stomach 30–1
stratum basale 67
stratum corneum 67
stratum granulosum 67
stratum spinosum 67
Streptococcus
  mitis 250
  mutans 23, 250, 251
    alveolar osteitis 98
    asthma 182
  salivarius 250–1
  sanguinis 250
  sobrinus 250
  Streptococcus anginosus
    group 250
  viscosus 250
streptokinase 224
streptozotocin 164–5
striae of Retzius 14

stroke 204–5
  aphasia 83–4
  aspiration pneumonia 78
  bronchial obstruction 176
  diabetes 160
  prevention 160
stylohyoid ligament 47
stylohyoid muscle 46, 47
stylomandibular
  ligament 47
sublingual artery 91
sublingual salivary gland 74
  control of secretion 75
submandibular salivary
  gland 74
  control of secretion 75
submental artery 91
submucosa 67
substance P 261
sucrose 23
superior alveolar nerve 265
  block
    complications 279
    procedure 278
superior dental plexus 265
superior laryngeal nerve 272
suppressor cells 241
  cell-mediated
    response 240
suprahyoid muscles 46–7
  ligaments 47
  temporomandibular
    joint 48
swallowing 78–9
  clinical application 78–9
  dry mouth 77
  impaired 78
  phases 78, 80
  of saliva, difficulties in 77
sweating, gustatory 273
sympathetic nervous
  system 268–73
  ganglion and effector
    receptors 268
synaptic transmission 259
syncope 194–5
syphilis 271
systematic
  desensitization 274
systemic inflammatory
  response syndrome
  (SIRS) 248
systemic lupus
  erythematosus 248
systole 188, 189

T

T helper cells 241
  cell-mediated
    response 240
  hypersensitivity 247

T lymphocytes 208,
    210, 234
  cell-mediated
    response 240
  hypersensitivity 247
  types 241
tacrolimus 229
tardive dyskinesia 284–5
  denture wearing 285
taste sensation 272–3
teeth
  autotransplantation 101
  development,
    chronology 9
  eruption 8–9
    delayed 9
  extraction 276
    see also extraction socket
  formation 2
    initiation stage 3
    stages 4, 5
  innervation 261
  orthodontic
    movement 100–1, 295
  osteoporosis 106
  see also permanent teeth;
    primary teeth
teething 8–9
telavancin 139
telomerase 109–10
temporalis muscle 40, 41
  temporomandibular
    joint 48
temporomandibular
  disorders
  jaw reflexes 57
  treatment 50–1
temporomandibular
  joint (TMJ)
  movements 48–9
  muscles of
    mastication 40–2
  structure and
    function 48–9
temporomandibular
  ligament 48
tension zone, orthodontic
  tooth movement 100
testosterone 290
tetrabenazine 77
tetracyclines 99, 131, 139,
    283
thalassaemias 219
  screening 219
third molars see impacted
    third molars
thrombin time 221
  coagulation screen 221
thrombocytopenia 222
thrombocytopenic
  purpura 222
thromboembolism 192

thrombolytic
    medication 224
thymoglobulin 229
thymus 234
thyroglobulin 298
thyroid cancer 301
  goitre 300
thyroid gland 298–301
  anatomy 298
thyroid hormones 298
  regulation 298
thyroid stimulating hormone
    (TSH) 298
  hyperthyroidism 300
  hypothyroidism 300
  regulation 298
  role 299
thyrotoxicosis 248, 298
thyrotrophin releasing
    hormone (TRH) 298
  regulation 298
thyroxine (T4) 298, 299
  hypothyroidism 300
ticagrelor 224
tidal volume 174, 175
tirofiban 224
tissue fluid hydrostatic
    pressure 8–9
tissue types 229
tobacco smoking see
    smoking
tooth see teeth
tooth germ 2
tooth surface loss (TSL) 37
trabecular bone 108
trachea 170
transferrin 213
transforming growth
    hormone 8–9
transient ischaemic attack
    (TIA) 205
transient receptor
    potential vanilloid
    receptor subtype 1
    (TRPV1) 260–1
transplants 229
  bone marrow 226–7
  face 229
  kidney 145
  liver 126
  stem cell see stem cell
    transplantation
  teeth 101
transtheoretical model
  of behavioural
  change 274
trauma, and pulpal
  pathology 243
Treponema 250
  denticola 98
β-tricalcium phosphate
  grafts 96

tricyclic antidepressants 269
trigeminal nerve (cranial
    nerve V) 266
  facial and dental pain 260
  facial skin sensation 264–5
  jaw reflexes 56–7
  mandibular division 264
  maxillary division 264–5
  muscles of
      mastication 40–2, 46
  nuclei 53
trigeminal neuralgia 56, 263
triiodothyronine
    (T3) 298, 299
trismus 278
trochlear nerve (cranial
    nerve IV) 267
tropocollagen 87
trypsin 150
tumour necrosis factor
    (TNF) 233
  cytokines 12–13
tumour suppressor genes
    (TSGs) 70
tumours 56

U

ulcerative colitis 248
ulcers
  diabetic 165, 166
  oral 68–9
ultrasonic scalers
  cardiovascular implantable
      electronic devices 199
  as cause of disease 183
unloading reflex 56
upper airway obstruction
  causes 176
  signs 176–7
  treatment 176
uraemic toxins 146

V

vaccination 238

vagal stimulation (gut) 32
vagus nerve (cranial
    nerve X) 266
  speech production 82–4
  taste sensation 272, 273
variant Creutzfeldt–
    Jakob disease
    (vCJD) 254–5
variceal bleeding 122
vascular defects 222–4
vascular dementia 205
vasoactive intestinal peptide
    (VIP) 292
  and somatostatin 302–3
vasopressin see antidiuretic
    hormone
Veillonella 23, 250
ventilation/perfusion (V/P)
    ratio 174
Ventolin 182
ventricular
    hypertrophy 179
verapamil 200
vertebrobasilar
    ischaemia 272
vestibulocochlear nerve
    (cranial nerve VIII) 266
viral infections 246
viruses 251
vital capacity 174
  forced see forced vital
      capacity
vitamin D
  bone 92, 93
  chronic kidney
      disease 144, 148
  chronic renal failure 138
  secondary hyperpara-
      thyroidism 93
vitamin K
  deficiency 223–4
  intravenous 130–1
vitamin K antagonist
    anti-coagulants 200
vitamins 35
vocalization 82–4

vomiting (emesis) 32–3
  eating disorders 37
  inhalation sedation 185
von Willebrand's
    disease 222–3

W

warfarin
  binding with plasma
      proteins 116
  blood clotting
      impairment 224
  cardiovascular
      disease 200
  chronic renal
      failure 138–9
  drug interactions 224,
      283
  international normalized
      ratio 221
  prothrombin time 221
  vitamin K deficiency 223–4
water lines, dental
    unit 255
Whipple's procedure 151
white blood cells
    (leucocytes) 208, 210
  formation 212–14
  malignancy 226–7
working side of the
    mandible 49
woven bone 89–91, 98–9
  diabetes 164

X

xerostomia see dry mouth

Z

Z-discs 61
zoledronic acid 139
zygomatic branch, trigeminal
    nerve 265
Zygomycetes 166–7